WITHDRAWN

NAVIGATING AAC

Speech and Language Therapists are assumed to have a knowledge of AAC (Augmentative and Alternative Communication). The reality is that, unless they have had a student clinical placement in this field, they will qualify with very little experience in this area.

This book is an approachable guide to AAC and covers the various types, including paper-based and voice-output communication aids. There is guidance on how to assess a person who might need AAC, and how to work collaboratively with those who support the person on a daily basis. The author discusses the importance of core vocabulary alongside a personalised vocabulary. There are pointers for referring to specialised services, signposting families to alternative sources of funding, and making a business case for buying AAC equipment.

Written by an expert in the field, this book provides tips and strategies for SLTs who are brand new to AAC, as well as experienced clinicians wanting to gain further confidence in working with this varied client group.

Alison Battye is the author of *Who's Afraid of AAC?* (2017). She is also a Specialist SLT in AAC and manager of regional specialised AAC services.

Navigating Speech and Language Therapy

Navigating the field of speech and language therapy can seem overwhelming to students and newly qualified therapists. This series is designed to provide concise, entry level summaries of key areas in speech and language therapy, providing a basic insight into a specific area of therapy. Comprising practical advice and guidance from an expert in the field, the books cover topics such as assessment, therapy, psychological approaches and onward referral. This is a useful tool for anyone new to speech and language therapy, or building confidence in their field.

NAVIGATING AAC

50 ESSENTIAL STRATEGIES AND RESOURCES FOR USING AUGMENTATIVE AND ALTERNATIVE COMMUNICATION

Alison Battye

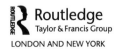
Routledge
Taylor & Francis Group
LONDON AND NEW YORK

2264

KH

First published 2023
by Routledge
4 Park Square, Milton Park, Abingdon, Oxon OX14 4RN

and by Routledge
605 Third Avenue, New York, NY 10158

Routledge is an imprint of the Taylor & Francis Group, an informa business

British Library Cataloguing-in-Publication Data
A catalogue record for this book is available from the British Library

ISBN: 978-1-032-28440-8 (hbk)
ISBN: 978-1-032-28441-5 (pbk)
ISBN: 978-1-003-29685-0 (ebk)

DOI: 10.4324/9781003296850

Typeset in Aldus
by Apex CoVantage, LLC

Thank you

Jane Madeley, who gave me the opportunity to write this book.

Karen Erickson and David Koppenhaver, for inspiring work on literacy development in the AAC world.

Georgina Overell and Nicola Fairburn, for your input into Chapter 5.

Marcin Zielonka, who has taken forward literacy and AAC in our service. Chapters 38 and 39 are indebted to your work.

My colleagues at KM CAT for inspiring me every day with the incredible work you do.

AAC users everywhere for setting the AAC agenda and insisting on being heard.

Stephen, Cate, Amelie and Kitty. Special thanks to Cate for your illustrations.

CONTENTS

LIST OF FIGURES

WHAT IS AAC?

AAC (Augmentative and Alternative Communication) describes a range of techniques and resources that can help someone to express themselves when their speech is difficult. It might augment their unclear speech, or it may be an alternative to speech if they have no natural voice.

In addition to supporting speech, AAC can also support a person's attention and listening, receptive language, expressive language, cognition and memory.

This book will set out the most common techniques and resources that might be used.

People who might benefit from AAC have diverse conditions and needs. They can include children or adults who have:

- Developmental disorders, like Down Syndrome, Autism Spectrum Disorder (ASD), global delay or learning disabilities.
- Conditions which affect sensory or motor functions, like Cerebral Palsy (CP).
- Degenerative conditions such as Muscular Dystrophy, Motor Neurone Disease (MND) or Multiple Sclerosis (MS).
- Temporary speech loss due to illness, surgery to the head or neck, or a traumatic brain injury, including stroke.

However this is not a definitive list. There will be additional circumstances whereby an individual will benefit from AAC. There will also be individuals with these conditions who do not need AAC.

The need for AAC can be very emotive. Our speech is part of our identity. Having a voice, and having natural speech, is highly valued in our culture.

For most people, natural speech is much easier and quicker than communicating using AAC. Natural speech produces over 125 words per minute. Once we have learnt to speak, we don't really have to think about selecting the right words, putting them in order, and making the correct speech sounds.

Communicating using AAC is slow: between 1 and 8 words per minute. It is also more effortful. AAC users and their communication partners have to put a lot of thought into vocabulary selection and how to create meaningful phrases, be it through signs, symbols or text. If the AAC user has physical disabilities or sensory loss, then there may be additional fatigue, because the AAC may be accessed using an alternative method, like switch-scanning or eye-pointing.

Therefore, a Speech and Language Therapist (SLT) needs to be skilled in introducing the topic of AAC.

Some questions to think about when considering whether an individual might need AAC are:

- Can they make their basic wants and needs known using natural speech?
- Can they communicate successfully with a range of people, familiar and unfamiliar?
- Are they getting frustrated because they cannot make themselves understood?
- Are their communication difficulties having an impact on their wellbeing?

If the answer is 'yes' to these questions, then you are reading the right book!

WHO IS THIS BOOK FOR?

This book is intended to serve as an introduction to AAC. You might be an SLT student, a recently qualified SLT, or a generalist SLT with little experience in AAC. You may specialise in another clinical area, but you need to know about a few AAC approaches. You may be returning to practice. You may be developing a specialism in AAC. You may work within health, education or social care, or you may be in independent practice.

The most commonly used resources and techniques are covered. You may dip in and out, identify particular chapters to read, or read the book in its entirety.

The book is divided into sections, which are:

- **Assessing for AAC**: this includes language assessment and specific AAC assessment, including how the person might access AAC.
- **Supporting the AAC user**: this includes key concepts for successful implementation and the most useful techniques for communication partners.
- **AAC solutions**: this includes the most common AAC solutions, including paper-based and screen-based solutions.
- **Building language skills with AAC**: this includes how to support vocabulary, sentence-building, and the social use of language.
- **Literacy, learning and AAC**: this includes the importance of literacy, an SLT's role in literacy teaching and access to the curriculum.
- **Advocacy and AAC**: this includes how we enable people to organise and express their thoughts and feelings about their care, and how AAC might support safeguarding and Mental Capacity assessment.
- **AAC and access to the world**: this includes how AAC might be integrated with Environmental control and social media, and how we promote AAC use in the wider world.
- **Funding for AAC**: this includes referral to specialist AAC services, and funding for AAC resources, for individuals and for SLT services.

The chapters are deliberately short. Each chapter will cover the essential information about a particular AAC solution or approach: what the approach is, its key features, the reason it helps, and who it is intended for. There are often 'next steps', and in many chapters there is a case study to help you apply theory to practice. Where appropriate, chapters include a 'Recommended resources' section where you can find more information. Where there are natural links between chapters, for example between communication partner training and conversation club, this is highlighted, so that you can flick between chapters.

At the end of the book is a chapter on continuing professional development. Here you can find recommended training, books, websites, blogs and 'Communication Matters', the charity for AAC users, which has an online AAC Forum, where you can post any questions and receive a reply from AAC experts.

ASSESSING
FOR AAC

2

HOW TO INTRODUCE
THE IDEA OF AAC

ESTABLISH A RELATIONSHIP FIRST

Before you can broach the topic of AAC, you will need to establish trust with the individual and their family. You will need to explain your role in supporting with communication. It is good practice to consult with them about the problem as they see it, and what they would like to change about their experiences of communication.

Areas to explore are:

- Can everyone understand you all of the time?
- What situations are difficult?
- Who with? Where? When?

Once you have a clearer idea of the problem, you can offer some hope that you may be able to help. You may already have some ideas about which forms of AAC may help. You may need to go away and do some thinking. Be open and honest about this: we all need time for thinking and researching the best solution for an individual.

AA WHAT?

Most people will not have heard of AAC. The term 'Augmentative and Alternative Communication' is not terribly enlightening.

DOI: 10.4324/9781003296850-3

SHOW THEM WHAT YOU MEAN

An easier way to introduce AAC may be to show a resource that you are thinking of trying. You may have the AAC resource available to demonstrate.

Alternatively, you may show a video of a person using the particular AAC resource. Communication Matters, CALL Scotland and the ACE Centre websites are good places to search for videos of people using AAC.

RESISTANCE TO AAC

Be prepared for a certain amount of resistance.

If you are working with children, then their parent or carer will be confronted with the possibility that speech will not develop as quickly as they had hoped. They may interpret your suggestion of using AAC as you giving up on their child's speech.

If you are working with adults with an acquired or degenerative condition, they will find it difficult to contemplate needing an alternative to speech.

WE ARE NOT GIVING UP ON SPEECH

Depending on the individual's circumstances, it will be worth stressing that you are not giving up on their speech. AAC has been shown to support speech development in children and young people.[1]

There is a fine balance between being realistic and allowing the individual and their family hope. If you are working with a child or young person, there is always hope that speech will develop.

Clinical experience suggests that AAC supports speech development in the following ways:

- AAC builds the foundations for speech, including attention and listening, receptive language and expressive language.

- AAC offers a visual support for the representation of language. AAC can physically show the structure of words and sentences, using symbols or text.
- It slows communication partners down, so that they do not overwhelm a person who needs longer to process spoken language.
- Voice Output Communication Aids (VOCAs) offer a highly consistent speech model which is very helpful for those who struggle to process speech sounds.

A TEMPORARY MEASURE

AAC can bridge a gap when a person has a temporary impairment due to illness, surgery or acquired brain injury. You can be honest about not knowing at this stage how long AAC will be needed. It will reduce frustration in the meantime.

DEGENERATIVE CONDITIONS

Degenerative conditions are perhaps the hardest to manage. You may be introducing the idea that there will be a time that the person will not be able to communicate their basic needs using speech, and this is incredibly confronting. This is emotional for you too, and you are likely to need support from colleagues when dealing with this situation. If this is your first time, then practise what you are going to say. Have strategies to deal with your own emotions in the session[2], so that you can help the individual and their family with theirs.

SAY WHAT AAC WILL OFFER

You are suggesting AAC because it will help to solve a problem the individual is having now or may have in the future. The exact way AAC might help will vary from individual to individual. Here are some possible ways AAC might help:

- It reduces the 'guess-work' which may be going on at the moment.

- It may add to the person's repertoire of total communication skills. AAC adds to the use of eye-contact, facial expressions, body language, gesture, pointing, eye-pointing, vocalisations and speech.
- It may allow the person to communicate about a wider range of topics. It can help cue a communication partner into a topic when they are struggling to understand a person's speech.
- It may allow the person to communicate with a wider range of people in different settings.
- It may allow the person to use a wider variety of communication functions, beyond basic requesting. For example, they could share their ideas, thoughts and feelings.
- It may provide a wider vocabulary and allow the person to use more sophisticated language. This may help them to convey their personality and ability to others.
- It may help the person to build on or make use of their literacy skills. Being able to give an initial letter in a word can really help others to guess an unclear word, for example when the person is talking about a person or place.

ACKNOWLEDGE THE CHALLENGES

Whilst it is important that you 'sell' the idea of AAC to the individual and their family, it is equally important that you acknowledge the feelings that come up for them. This may be spoken or unspoken. They may include:

- Grief for the loss of speech, or loss of hope for straightforward development of speech.
- Fear about looking different. We live in a disablist society and see different as bad.
- Overwhelm about learning a new set of skills. AAC is a whole new communication mode, and new strategies need to be learnt.
- Fear about what the future holds. You cannot offer false hope, but you can offer to be present with them.

OFFER THINKING TIME

If an individual or their family resists AAC, offer some thinking time so that you can come back to it. As human beings we often resist a new idea when it is first suggested. You may agree a timeframe for coming back to the discussion.

WHERE THERE ARE DISAGREEMENTS

If you think that the person themselves would benefit from AAC but that their family or carers are resisting it, you may need to carry out a Mental Capacity Assessment (see Chapter 42).

If you have concerns that carers may be restricting a person's right to communication, you will need to contact your safeguarding team.

CASE STUDY: ABDI'S NEED FOR AAC

Abdi had a stroke which affected his word-finding. He tends to make semantic errors, saying a word from the same category. He can no longer read, but he can make good attempts to spell a word.

When the SLT suggested that Abdi might want to use a pen and paper alongside his speech, he didn't feel this was needed. He was managing at home with his partner, Gordon. However, Gordon felt that Abdi was getting depressed because he was not venturing out anymore. Abdi had stopped going out with his walking club because he was embarrassed when he couldn't communicate at cafes.

Abdi agreed to try using a notepad. He and Gordon practised at their local shops over the next week. They also tried using the notes app on Abdi's phone and found that this was even better, because the prediction feature for spelling words sped up Abdi's rate of typing. He was able to type longer messages and had even shared a joke with his pharmacist.

> Abdi reflected that he could use the notes app to pre-
> pare messages for people who he knew he was going to
> see. He emailed his old walking club friend and was going
> to try a short walk at the weekend. Gordon felt that there
> was less pressure on him to support Abdi's communica-
> tion, and that they both had more independence.

NOTES

1 Millar, D., Light, J. and Schlosser, R. 'The impact of augmentative
  and alternative communication intervention on the speech production of individuals with developmental disabilities: a research
  review', *Journal of Speech, Language, and Hearing Research*,
  2006, Apr; 49(2):248–64.
2 For example, you might like to explore chapters about resilience
  and adversity in the author's previous book: Battye, A. *Self-Care
  for Allied Health Professionals: From Surviving to Thriving*,
  Routledge, 2021.

EVERYONE ON BOARD

Whilst you may be the person who introduces the idea of AAC and takes the lead in choosing the most appropriate solution, you will need a team alongside you. An AAC solution cannot be established by an SLT alone. Nor can it be implemented and maintained by an SLT alone.

Your team will include:

- The AAC user
- Family, friends and carers
- Professionals working with the AAC user

Anyone who regularly communicates with the person using AAC has a role to play in its implementation.

CONVINCING THE POTENTIAL AAC USER

The person themself will need to be on board with using AAC. This is generally easy with children, who tend to be highly adaptable. If the child has good receptive language but for some reason has not developed speech, then they will likely embrace AAC communication, because it is their first experience of expressive language. If their receptive language is impaired, then they may welcome the visual support that AAC brings. This may open up the world of spoken language for them. So long as the first few trials are fun, unpressurised and anything they say is accepted as meaningful, they are likely to go with it.

For children and adults who have not yet developed joint attention and communicative intent, you may need to work on

DOI: 10.4324/9781003296850-4

this before you introduce AAC. See Chapter 6 on developing the foundations for AAC.

For children, young people and adults who have some speech or who have lost speech, AAC communication is likely to be less appealing. It is different; it is slow; it requires a lot of effort to learn. As the SLT you can acknowledge this.

Sometimes those around the potential AAC user have protected them from knowing how unintelligible their speech is. This may be the time for gentle honesty. Communication partners may need to say when they don't understand, otherwise the potential AAC user will see no need for AAC.

THE FIRST TRIALS OF AAC

The first exposure to AAC will need to be fun and meaningful. You might arrange it so that the first tries are 'error free'. You might set up a page of vocabulary around a motivating topic, for example, people, pets, or favourite places. You might ask them to tell you about their favourite food, animal, place or activity. The initial topic might naturally move on to related topics, so that you can demonstrate more pages of vocabulary.

As an SLT, you have the communication skills to help the individual to repair any mistakes or miscommunication. Use your observations of their multi-modal communication, especially their facial expressions and body language, to help you identify when the message was not completely successful. AAC communication involves shared creation of meaning. The communication partner needs to work harder to add nuances or personal references for that AAC user.

FAMILY, FRIENDS AND CARERS

The potential AAC user may take their lead from those around them. Never underestimate the power of communication partners in conveying positive or negative messages about AAC!

If you are sensing resistance, ask them about this. Try to create a relationship where they can be open and honest. If you get negative feedback about the AAC system, take a moment to process what they have said before you respond. Come back to the reasons you believed AAC would be helpful in Chapter 2.

Acknowledge that no AAC solution is as fast and automatic as speech, but that speech currently needs supporting.

Remind them that whilst they might be able to understand the person, not everyone can. And no one, not even a parent or a partner, can anticipate exactly what another person is thinking all of the time.

If the AAC user has mental capacity, then it is their choice whether they use AAC, and any carers need to respect this.

It may be useful to demonstrate the AAC user's skills by videoing them using their AAC system and having this video available to any paid carers. Communication passports are also a good way to give instructions to new staff. (See Chapter 30.)

PROFESSIONALS WORKING WITH THE AAC USER

The potential AAC user is likely to have a team of professionals already involved. There may also be a need to make additional referrals.

Not all AAC users will need all of the professionals listed below. If the AAC user does not have physical or sensory disabilities, the team around them will be smaller.

- Occupational Therapists provide advice and equipment to support posture and seating, and the best access method for an individual. See Chapter 8 for more information about assessing for access method.
- Physiotherapists also provide input for posture and movement. Refer to local criteria for physiotherapy and occupational therapy input regarding AAC.
- If there is sensory impairment, you will need to involve the VI or HI Specialist.
- If the AAC user is a child or young person, then teaching staff, including teachers and teaching assistants are going to play a central role in effective AAC implementation. You

will need to set objectives jointly for access to the curriculum, as well as social communication with peers.

- If the AAC user has physical or sensory disabilities, they may also access Wheelchair or Environmental Controls services. If you are considering an AAC solution which requires mounting on a wheelchair, or integrating with environmental controls (to control doors or lights or electrical devices in the home), then you will need to involve these services.

This all requires good communication! You might arrange a professionals meeting: I can't emphasise enough the importance of everyone being in the same room. It ensures that everyone gets heard, can express their concerns from the start, and can be part of the solution. Of course, the AAC user and their immediate support team are fundamental to this, so they will also need to attend.

The roles to be agreed might include:

- Assessment of access methods (likely to be an OT or Physiotherapist).
- Assessment of speech, language and communication skills (see Chapter 5).
- Creation of the AAC solution, be it paper-based or computer or tablet-based.
- Supporting AAC communication every day, throughout the day. Everyone is involved in this. You, as the SLT, will need to model AAC skills (see Chapter 11) or provide some level of training for others (see Chapter 12).
- Updating of the vocabulary. A child's vocabulary is constantly growing. An adult may start new activities, or their circumstances will change so that they need different words and phrases. You will need some way of adding words. This is not entirely the responsibility of the SLT, but you need to provide guidance about how to organise vocabulary. Ideally, we want to empower the AAC user's immediate support team to be able to add vocabulary themselves.

- Ongoing maintenance of the AAC. If a computer or tablet-based device is used, someone will need to charge it, inspect it for safety and carry out any software updates. Ideally this will be someone in the AAC user's immediate family or who sees them every day.

It can be very useful to draw up an action plan, stating who will do what. Having something written down that you can refer to can hold people accountable. If a person is not doing what they said they would, then at least you have a starting point for discussion and negotiation. Often just reminding people of what they signed up to is enough of a prompt. You may need to remind people of the benefit of AAC. (see 'Say what AAC will offer' in Chapter 2).

EXAMPLE ACTION PLAN

Action:	Responsibility:
Assess functional vision, with different symbol and text sizes and arrays.	OT
Assess receptive language and use Frenchay screening tool to assess need for symbols or text.	SLT
Complete vocabulary checklist to supply relevant names of people and pets, favourite activities, etc.	Bernie and Carer
Begin communication book template, once the above has been submitted. Share and discuss with Bernie and carer.	SLT

GET TO KNOW THE PERSON

No two human beings are the same, so no two AAC users are going to be the same. In order to develop a 'good fit' AAC solution, you are going have to get to know them.

There is a danger in AAC assessment that we simply see a diagnosis, or a list of clinical strengths and needs. Of course it is important that we understand the person's clinical needs (we will explore this more in the next chapter), but first and foremost, they are a person with a unique identity. We need to honour this.

IDENTITY

Communication is not a simple exchange to get our basic needs met. Communication is more profound: it is the way we relate to others and connect with others. In order to fully connect, we need to feel that the other person acknowledges and honours our identity.

Our identity is made up of our personality and our interests. It is also made up of socially created roles. These encompass gender, sexuality, race, ethnicity, age, social class, family background, educational background, work experiences, health, disability, sub-culture identifications and so on. Our relationships come into play: whether we are a partner, a parent, daughter, son, sister, brother, and so on. Our profession, religion or sporting affiliations may be more or less important to us at different stages in our life.

It is important that any AAC solution reflects our identity. We will need to think about the vocabulary and phrasing within the AAC solution. We will need to consider the physical appearance of the AAC solution. If there is to be voice-output,

DOI: 10.4324/9781003296850-5

then we need to work closely with the AAC user so that they feel that the voice is a good match for them.

HOW DO WE FIND OUT ABOUT THIS?

It may at first seem awkward or intrusive to ask questions about identity, but if you explain why you are asking (to get a full picture of them as a person in order to find the best-fit AAC solution), people are generally happy to engage.

Some questions that you might ask of the AAC user or of their family or carers include:

- What lights you up?
- What would your perfect day look like?
- Who are you closest to?
- What roles have you played in your life (professional, voluntary)?
- Do you belong to any groups or clubs?
- Do you speak other languages?
- Have you travelled?
- What music do you love listening to?
- Who do you admire?

COMMUNICATION CONTEXTS

We want to know all about how the AAC user communicates now, and how they would like to communicate in the future. This is not only about them expressing their wants and needs. We are aiming for them to feel emotionally connected to others, to be able to convey their personality and co-create rich social meanings from their exchanges.

We might ask:

- Who will they communicate with?
- Where will they be? Will it be noisy or busy? How are they moving around?
- Will they be on their own or accompanied by a carer?
- What do they want and need to communicate?

- What other communication functions might they need (greeting, giving information, asking and answering questions, giving their opinion, describing, telling stories, reporting a concern, repairing communication breakdowns, negotiating, expressing feelings, expressing closeness)?
- Why do they want or need to do this (independence, safety, physical or emotional wellbeing)?
- How would they like to do it? (What mode of communication?)

These questions do not have to be answered all at once. We don't want to reduce them to a tick sheet. Some of them may unfold as you get to know a person. Certain questions may become more relevant at particular points in your assessment of intervention.

The important thing is that we are receptive to messages about the person's unique identity and communication contexts. We show cultural curiosity when we are learning about their circumstances, and we involve them in decisions about their AAC solution, because it is going to make up an important part of their identity.

ASSESS, DON'T GUESS!

RECEPTIVE LANGUAGE LEVEL

I can't emphasise enough the importance of knowing someone's receptive language level. In order to provide a good AAC system to support their expressive language, we need to know how much they understand.

FORMAL ASSESSMENTS

You may use formal assessments if these are accessible for the person. Formal assessments tend to be comprehensive but extremely lengthy. It is often more appropriate to choose selected sub-tests only for a person with physical, sensory or cognitive impairment.

For children and adults, the TROG-2[1] is useful. It is fairly quick to administer but gives a lot of information about their receptive language.

For adults, you may use parts of the PALPA.[2] Try to narrow down your assessment so that you are only using the sub-test that is most clinically relevant to them.

MAKING ASSESSMENT MATERIALS ACCESSIBLE

If the person cannot finger-point, you may need to space the pictures out so that they can fist-point.

You might wish to point to each picture in turn, saying 'Is it this one?' and wait for them to indicate a yes or no (see Chapter 22 for Partner-Assisted Auditory Scanning).

For someone who can eye-point, you may place the picture materials on an E-Tran frame (see Chapter 23).

INFORMAL RECEPTIVE LANGUAGE ASSESSMENT: INFORMATION-CARRYING WORDS

If you cannot carry out a formal receptive language assessment, or part of a formal assessment, or if the person has limited attention, then you can still assess their receptive language level informally.

It is really helpful to know how many information-carrying words a person can understand. This will help you to train communication partners to use the right level of language for the person. It will also help you to design an AAC solution at the right level of receptive language.

Below is a suggestion for assessing information-carrying words, but you might also use a tool like the Derbyshire Rapid Screening Test.[3] Make sure that this is accessible for the individual. In the examples below, the person would need good vision, including colour vision. They would also need to be familiar with these cultural concepts. You may choose to adapt the concepts according to the person's experiences.

1 INFORMATION-CARRYING WORD

Without giving the person any clues in your tone of voice or what you are looking at, can they point to:

- A named noun from a choice of four nouns (e.g. cat, dog, chair, table)?
- A named verb from a choice of four verbs (e.g. eating, drinking, sitting, standing)?

2 INFORMATION-CARRYING WORDS

Can they point to a picture from a choice of four showing:

- A noun and verb (e.g. cat eating, cat sleeping, dog eating, dog sleeping)? For every information-carrying word, there needs to be a contrast.
- An adjective and a noun (e.g. big cup, little cup, big spoon, little spoon)?

3 INFORMATION-CARRYING WORDS

Can they point to a picture from a choice of four similar options showing:

- A combination of adjective, noun and verb (e.g. cat sleeping on a chair, dog sleeping on a chair, cat standing on a chair, cat sleeping on a table)?
- A combination of adjective, noun and preposition (e.g. big ball on the box, big ball in the box, little ball on the box, big ball on the table)?

HOW DOES THIS HELP YOU?

If the person does not understand 1 information-carrying word, we need to use pointing, signs and symbols to support spoken language.

If they understand 1 information-carrying word, we can support longer spoken instructions with pointing, or using signs or symbols. We need to 'chunk' information so that we do not overwhelm the person. All those who communicate with the person need to know this. We will model mainly single words when we use this person's AAC, but we may sometimes model more. They may have a simple communication board with 'core' words (high-frequency words which are useful in all situations), or a simple communication book with core words and a few pages of 'fringe' words (see Chapters 17 and 31).

A person who understands 2 information-carrying words can cope with us using 2–3 information-carrying words in a phrase, as long as these are supported with AAC. Their AAC system will need to allow for combining words into phrases. They will probably be ready for a book, rather than a board, to provide more language.

A person who understands 3 or more information-carrying words will need even more language. They will need an AAC solution which has many pages of vocabulary that allows them to combine words into phrases.

An adult with good receptive language and literacy levels may be able to build their own sentences from scratch, either spelling words using an alphabet chart, or choosing words from an array. They may also have a list of commonly used phrases to choose from.

PHOTOS, PICTURES, SYMBOLS OR TEXT?

In addition to assessing receptive language, you will also need to know if the person can recognise photos, pictures, symbols or text.

Photos and pictures are limiting. For nouns, you need a clear background for the noun to stand out. The noun needs to be generic enough to represent that concept even if the colour or size differs. Verbs, adjectives and prepositions are not easy to represent in photos. Line drawings and pictures are similarly tricky.

This is why symbols are useful. If a person can understand symbols, then use symbols rather than photos or pictures. There are established symbol sets like Widgit Literacy Symbols, Picture Communication Symbols and Symbolstix. These are designed to be as clear and easily interpreted as possible. See Chapter 37 for more information on recommended symbol sets.

If a person can read, then text is even better. A symbol vocabulary is limited by the person choosing the vocabulary. It cannot possibly include every possible concept a person will need. An alphabet chart or keyboard offers an unlimited number of words. It even allows the person to create new words: something that we love to do as human beings. Check that a person is not only decoding words, but also able to access the meaning of the word. A picture-to-text matching test[4] will help establish this if there is any doubt.

If we are considering a computer- or tablet-based AAC solution, then prediction software within a text-to-speech app can speed up a person's rate of typing. The AAC user may only need to type the first two or three letters and then choose the whole word from the prediction options.

SPECIFIC AAC ASSESSMENT TOOLS

There are some specific AAC assessment tools which may help you narrow down your decisions about the specific AAC solution which meets a person's needs. These are informal tests, and not all sections need to be administered.

The Test of Aided Communication Performance (TASP)[5] assesses for the symbol size and number of symbols per page that the person can access. It also assesses their categorisation skills and some syntax and grammatical abilities.

The Frenchay Screening Tool for AAC[6] assesses for physical access, visual processing and acuity for the symbol size and number of symbols per page, text size and categorisation. It also assesses reading with and without symbol support, sentence-to-picture matching and paragraph reading and comprehension. It goes on to assess for spelling and coding.

Both of these assessments can be used with children and adults. Of the two assessments, the Frenchay is the most comprehensive.

CASE STUDY: LEONIE'S LEVEL OF UNDERSTANDING

Leonie has a very sociable nature, and loves being at school.

School staff feel that Leonie understands everything. She smiles and laughs when they make jokes. She also complies with all their suggestions for activities. They feel that she doesn't need AAC because she never gets frustrated.

The SLT carried out an informal assessment of Leonie's receptive language and found that she was understanding at a 1 information-carrying word level. She did not yet understand verbs, adjectives or prepositions.

School staff were surprised, but on reflection, they realised that they were supporting Leonie's receptive language with a lot of Makaton signing and gesture, as well as their non-verbal communication. She was very adept at picking up on their facial expressions and laughter, and she copied these.

The SLT stressed that he still wanted staff to support Leonie's understanding in this way, using Makaton signs and showing what they meant when they were talking. They were also to introduce symbols in the form a communication book. The SLT showed them how to use the core words, which were on each page, and fringe words, which were specific to the topic. They could use core words in any activity, e.g. 'more', 'stop', 'go', 'want', 'like', 'open', 'help', 'you', 'here' and 'on'. They could also model a few two-word phrases, like 'want it' and 'you help' (core words only) and 'look bird' and 'car go' (core and fringe).

When Leonie's receptive language was assessed again twelve months later, she was consistently understanding 2 information-carrying words, including verbs. Expressively, Leonie was starting to combine two symbols in a phrase.

NOTES

1 Test for the Reception of Grammar 2 (TROG-2) by Dorothy Bishop, Pearson Clinical, 2003.

2 Psycholinguistic Assessments of Language Processing in Aphasia (PALPA) by Janice Kay, Max Coltheart and Ruth Lesser, Psychology Press, 1992.

3 Derbyshire Rapid Screening Test, Derbyshire Language Scheme.

4 For children, use downloadable resources on sites like Twinkl. Search 'word to picture matching' or 'sentence to picture matching'. For adults, you may use: 'letter length reading' (PALPA 29), 'letter length spelling' (PALPA 39), 'spoken word to picture

matching' (PALPA 47), 'written word to picture matching' (PALPA 48) and the 'written sentence comprehension' (PALPA 56).

5 Test of Aided-Communication Symbol Performance (TASP) by Joan Bruno, Boardmaker Products.

6 Frenchay Screening Tool for AAC, Logan Technologies.

THE FOUNDATIONS FOR AAC

There are certain developmental stages and associated skills that must be in place for communication to progress. These are the same for AAC as they are for verbal communication.

Human beings are social animals. We have an innate desire to connect with one another. We need other people to 'get' us. It starts with joint attention.

JOINT ATTENTION

Joint attention is the ability for a child to focus on the same thing as an adult in order to enjoy interaction together.

Initially joint attention just involves two people. For instance, a baby and caregiver gazing at one another and copying facial expressions or vocalisations. This happens more or less from birth in typically developing infants. Sensory, physical or cognitive impairment may interfere with this.

If an individual is very much in their own world and not apparently seeking communication, an approach called intensive interaction[1] is a great place to start. The communication partner meets them where they are at, noticing what they are interested in. The communication partner copies what the individual does, in order to get their attention and to build a shared moment.

In typical development, joint attention extends to include an outside focus of interest. This is 'three-way' joint attention. They might be looking at something together, say a dog or a picture book. Both the adult and the child are focused on this interesting thing, and they are sharing a moment together. They might look at one another and then back at the dog.

 DOI: 10.4324/9781003296850-7

This three-way joint attention starts to develop at around six months for a typically developing child.

Attention is fleeting at first: any interruption, like a new person walking into the room, will completely re-set the child's attention. With time, the child can focus for longer, and can maintain focus even in the face of visual or auditory distractions.

Joint attention is important for AAC because we are asking the AAC user to modulate their attention between a person, a topic of conversation, and the AAC itself. Makaton signs can help before three-way attention has developed, because they draw attention to the communication partner. If the individual has developed three-way joint attention, then symbols can be introduced.

COMMUNICATIVE INTENT

Communicative intent is the desire to communicate.

Before communicative intent has developed, an individual is described as 'pre-intentional'. They do not consciously communicate in order to convey a particular message. An example would be a newborn baby crying. They do not initially cry with the knowledge that someone will come and pick them up. With experience, they learn that this does often happen. They know that crying or shouting will result in an adult coming, and so they will consciously make noise to get attention. This is intentional communication, or communicative intent.

Communicative intent is related to 'cause-and-effect' understanding. Cause-and-effect understanding is the understanding that 'when I do A, then B happens'. For example, when I drop a cup, it makes a noise. Cause-and-effect understanding emerges at around nine months for a typically developing child. It develops into social understanding of cause-and-effect, for example when I shout, the adult turns to look at me. Cause-and-effect may not have a social element, but communicative intent is always social: the person has a message to convey to someone else. They may do this non-verbally or verbally, or with the support of AAC.

Communicative intent becomes more refined with frequent opportunities for interaction. The child learns that a specific behaviour leads to a particular response from adults. Shouting results in the adult stopping what they are doing. Vocalising and reaching for a book results in the adult bringing the book and sitting down to read a story together.

For some children, communicative intent may develop later than expected. Some adults with learning disabilities may not have developed communicative intent yet. Communication partners need to work hard at giving the person frequent opportunities to engage. They might need to experiment with different sensory experiences, interactive games or songs, in order to elicit a response from the individual. The communication partner needs to be tuned into subtle behaviours, such as facial expressions, body language or even breathing patterns, which signal that the person is interested. Any signal will be rewarded with interaction, and the repetition of the fun activity. The communication partner may then help to shape the behaviour into a more conventional communication behaviour. They may wait for the person to vocalise or look at them before the fun action is repeated.

AAC, in the form of single signs or symbols, may be introduced at this stage. The signs or symbols will probably represent the activity or the fun action that happens when the person has engaged. The communication partner might point to a symbol that says 'go!' or 'more!' as they blow bubbles or sing a song.

Soon there may be opportunities for choosing between two activities. Signs or symbols can be used to represent these choices. For example 'light tube' or 'swing'.

Making choices reinforces communicative intent. The individual learns that they consistently get the same response when they choose the symbol for 'ball' compared with 'bubbles'. Similarly, 'more' and 'stop' have very different results. This is the start of receptive language.

EXPERIENCE OF THE WORLD

To learn, we need to experience predictable patterns in the world.

We need to see, hear, touch, taste and smell the things in our environment to begin to understand what they are. Our sensory and motor outputs coordinate so that we can learn about the features and qualities of objects and how we might interact with them. We need some level of consistency to be able to associate particular actions with people, places and times in the day.

To learn language, we need repeated and consistent exposure to a word. Caregivers need to say the word just as we are giving it our attention.

For instance, the caregiver says 'ball' when the child is playing with the ball. They ideally do this several times, for as long as the child is interested in the ball.

For a child who is learning language using AAC, we need the communication partner to say 'ball' and to point at the symbol at the same time. This will help the child to understand the word 'ball' and that the symbol also refers to it.

A child with disabilities may have gaps in their experience of the world because they have not experienced such high levels of independent exploration. They may need more time to explore. They may need distant objects to be brought to them so that they can interact with them. They may need repeated exposure to the learning experience in order to make sense of it. They require a high level of consistency, so that different adults name the item in the same way, saying the word and pointing to the symbol.

CASE STUDY: BILLY'S FOUNDATIONS FOR AAC

Billy is five years old. Billy was ill as a baby and spent extended periods in hospital. He is now much more medically stable and beginning to show some interest in people and the world around him. It is possible that Billy has a cortical blindness, and this is under investigation.

Billy's parents notice that he loves noise-making toys and household objects which make a noise. He also loves his parents to sing and dance with him.

Billy's parents, in collaboration with his SLT, decide to focus on these activities.

They play a 'ready steady go' game, leaving a gap before they say 'go!' They wait for Billy to indicate he wants them to say 'go!' before they say it. They observe that he takes in an excited breath. This is their cue to say 'go!' Billy's parents position themselves face-to-face with him and notice that he has begun to look towards their faces when he anticipates them saying 'go!'

Because Billy missed so much time exploring the world around him, Billy's parents consciously let him explore household objects and show him the noises they make. He especially loves banging on pots and pans. Very soon he is waiting for them to say 'go!' before he bangs them.

NOTE

1   Hewett, D. (ed.) *The Intensive Interaction Handbook,* Second edition, Sage, 2018.

A CONSISTENT 'YES' OR 'NO'

A consistent 'yes' or 'no' response is crucial in AAC communication for the following reasons:

- It allows the communication partner to check that they are using strategies that are helping, e.g. 'Is this your communication book?' 'Do I read the options to you?'
- It allows the communication partner to check that they have correctly interpreted the message, e.g. 'Something about your partner. Do you want me to call them?'
- If the AAC system is not available, the communication partner can fall back on offering options and the AAC user responding with a 'yes' or 'no', e.g. 'Do you have pain in your: back? [pause] hips? [pause] shoulders?' [pause; AAC user indicates 'yes'].

A CONVENTIONAL 'YES' AND 'NO'

It is helpful if the AAC user has a conventional way to indicate 'yes' and 'no'. This means that their 'yes' and 'no' can be understood by unfamiliar communication partners.

The AAC user may be encouraged to indicate 'yes' and 'no' in any of the following conventional ways:

- Say an approximation of the word. Just the vowel sound is helpful.
- Nod their head for 'yes' and and shake their head for 'no'.
- Use a Makaton sign of a closed fist 'nodding' for 'yes', and an open palm swiping sideways for 'no'.

DOI: 10.4324/9781003296850-8

If none of these methods are available to the AAC user, then it may be that they:

- Wear 'yes' and 'no' wristbands.
- Look at 'yes' and 'no' symbols on different sides of their wheelchair tray.

I would suggest that right is 'yes' and left is 'no'. It will be important to be absolutely consistent in this, and possibly use colour-coding: green for 'yes' and red for 'no'.

CASE STUDY: THEO'S CONSISTENT 'YES' AND 'NO'

Theo had many different ways of saying 'yes' or 'no', but they were not consistent and not everyone agreed what they meant. One carer felt that he looked up for 'yes' and looked to the side for 'no'. Another carer said that he vocalised for 'yes' and sighed for 'no'.

After watching video of Theo, the team agreed that the vocalisation for 'yes' and the head-turning for 'no' were the easiest to understand. They agreed that they would ask Theo to 'tell me yes or no' when they were offering food, drinks, activities and so on. For the next week they tried to ask him frequent 'yes' or 'no' questions, and they would give him clear feedback about his response.

When the team met again, they reported that Theo was initially a bit confused, but quickly got the idea of signalling 'yes' and 'no' in the same way to every communication partner. In fact, he was now beginning to vocalise the vowel sound in 'no' too.

When Theo went to the café later that week, the staff understood his 'yes' and 'no' clearly, and Theo felt much more included in ordering his food.

TEACHING 'YES' AND 'NO'

For a person who does not yet understand the meaning of 'yes' and 'no', the communication partners will need to model it constantly. They will need to offer items throughout the day, using the same script: 'Do you want the ball? Yes or no?' They will then read the person's non-verbal signals, through their facial expression or body language. The communication partner will say 'yes! You want the ball!' or 'no. You don't want the ball.' Makaton signs will be helpful to accompany the words 'yes' and 'no' because the sign will draw attention to these words.

The communication partner will need to be attuned to the person's non-verbal signals. Mistakes can be a learning opportunity. If the person looks disappointed because the communication partner misinterpreted their response, then the communication partner can say 'I thought you said yes. You nodded like this.'

CASE STUDY: ANESHA'S 'YES' AND 'NO' TO CONFIRM OR CORRECT

Anesha is dependent on adults for all her care needs. She tends to be a 'people pleaser'. The team around her want her to be able to say when she doesn't like something: to be able to say a clear 'no'.

They start with funny questions. They pick up her shoe and say, 'Anesha, is this your hat?' and 'Shall we put this on your head?' They bring in other children to the activity who model saying 'no!' Anesha sees that this is fun and that it is ok to say 'no'. During play activities and reading, the adults ask the whole group 'is this a giraffe?' when they point to a picture of an elephant. The whole group, including Anesha, says or shakes their head 'no!'

Gradually, the team start asking Anesha if she wants to do certain activities, where some are more fun than others. For example, 'Anesha, would you like to sit here quietly whilst the others go out to play?' The staff member reminds Anesha 'you can say no!' Anesha shakes her head 'no'. She gets to go out and play with her friends.

Once the person is getting the hang of a 'yes' or 'no' to accept or reject an item or an activity, the communication partners can move on to asking other sorts of 'yes' and 'no' questions. They can also ask questions to check they have got something right, for example 'Is this your bag?' or 'Do you get the bus to school?'

When there is doubt that an AAC message has been correctly interpreted, the communication partner can say 'Was that right?' and 'Do you want to tell me more?'

Everyday communication using AAC is a great opportunity to practice 'yes' and 'no'. For instance:

- Do you have something to say?
- Do you need your communication book?
- Is it on this page?
- Did I get that right?
- Do want to tell me more?
- Anything else?

'YES' AND 'NO' QUESTIONS TO SHOW LEARNING

AAC users may struggle to answer open questions using their AAC, but if they have a clear 'yes' and 'no' a teacher can quickly assess their learning.

The teacher can ask a question and then use partner-assisted scanning to offer options. One of the options is the right answer. This is essentially a verbal multiple choice. For example, 'Tell me what letter the word "tap" starts with. Is it: "p", "d", "t", "b"?'

The options may be verbal, or they may be supported by pictures, symbols or written text. For example, 'Which one is a liquid? This one? This one? This one? This one?' Again the AAC user says 'yes' to the correct option.

ASSESSING FOR ACCESS METHOD

WHO ASSESSES FOR THE BEST ACCESS METHOD?

Occupational Therapists (OTs) are best placed to assess for the best way for a potential AAC user to access an AAC solution. OTs have expertise in fine motor skills, functional movement patterns, and postural supports and seating which facilitates this. OTs can carry out a functional vision assessment, if needed.

Other professionals who may be able to support this assessment include physiotherapists, VI or HI specialists, healthcare scientists and clinical technologists. Just like in speech and language therapy, different individuals have different skills sets and levels of experience. If it is unclear who should help you with this assessment, you will need to seek advice from your manager.

Sometimes the access method is straightforward: the AAC user may be able to finger-point, or press parts of a screen or keyboard easily. In this case, the role of the OT may be minimal. However, if physical disabilities, sensory impairment, coordination or fatigue are factors, then it is best to consult an OT or other relevant colleague for this part of the assessment process.

THE IMPORTANCE OF POSTURAL SUPPORT AND SEATING

Just like we need an optimum set-up in our workspace to avoid repetitive strain and eye-strain, we need to make sure that the AAC user has the optimum set-up of their AAC solution. This may involve angling the communication board, book or device

DOI: 10.4324/9781003296850-9

so that they can easily see it without craning their neck. They must be positioned so that they are able to point to or activate all areas of their AAC solution. This might involve the use of a tray or cushioned supports for their arms and wrists. If the AAC user has uncontrolled movements, then they may need AAC equipment to be velcroed to a tray or mounted on a wheelchair.

If the physical or sensory needs of the AAC user change, then they will need reassessment from the relevant professional. This is especially true for growing children or those who have degenerative conditions.

FUNCTIONAL VISION ASSESSMENT

If there is doubt over an AAC user's vision, you may need to request a Functional Vision Assessment. This can include near and far vision, the visual field, contrast sensitivity, colour vision, figure-ground perception, visual fixation and visual tracking. This will influence the size of text or symbols, their layout on a page or screen, and any colour contrasts that are needed.

There are local differences in how to access a functional vision assessment, and so you may need to make enquiries.

DIRECT SELECTION METHODS

Direct selection means that an AAC user can directly point to or activate their AAC solution. They may finger-point or fist-point to text or symbols on a page or press parts of a screen or keyboard. Some AAC users may benefit from a keyguard or a specialist dibber to improve the accuracy of their selections and prevent mis-hits.

If finger-pointing is not an option, other parts of the body may be recruited. They may use a head-pointer or head-mouse.

An AAC user may use a standard mouse or they may benefit from a specialist mouse like joystick, rollerball or glide-pad.

Eye-gaze technology may also enable direct selections. Eye-gaze cameras can either be mounted to a mainstream computer or may be integral to a dedicated AAC device. The camera picks up eye-movements and this translates into moving a cursor and making selection depending on dwell-time or a blink. This is a surprisingly tiring access method, and not many people cannot tolerate it. It takes time to learn the various skills needed to successfully use eye-gaze technology, including learning to fixate, track and time eye-movements.

INDIRECT SELECTION METHODS

If a person has physical disabilities affecting the accuracy of their movements, then partner-assisted scanning or switch-scanning may be a better option.

In partner-assisted scanning using paper-based AAC, the communication partner will read out options and the AAC user will indicate 'yes' to select the desired option. The most used items will be listed first, to cut down on the time that the AAC user needs to wait to get to the desired item. (For more on Partner-Assisted Auditory Scanning, see Chapter 22.)

In switch-scanning, a switch, or a small button, will be set up so that the AAC user can press the switch to make a selection on a screen. The switch site will depend upon the AAC user's most reliable voluntary movement. Head switches can be mounted onto a wheelchair head-rest. Switches can also be velcroed into position on a wheelchair tray or foot-rest.

The AAC user may just use one switch, in which case the device will be set up to automatically scan through options, and the AAC user will press the switch when it gets to the desired option. The scanning pattern may be row-column, or may highlight blocks of the screen in a particular order. This requires patience and good timing skills to activate the switch at the right time.

Alternatively, an AAC user may use two switches: one for moving a scanner on to the next item, and one for selecting the desired item. The scanning speed can also be individualised.

TIME TO DEVELOP ACCESS SKILLS

An OT will work with the AAC user to determine which access method works best, and skills may need to be built over time.

All those working with the AAC user will need to know how to set up the access equipment, and they will need to provide frequent opportunities to practice skills. A younger AAC user may practice these skills by playing simple computer games, like 'Big Bang' or 'Choose It!'. As their accuracy improves, they may be able to access an AAC vocabulary package or onscreen keyboard. Some AAC users can access an AAC vocabulary package or onscreen keyboard straight away.

Sometimes AAC users' needs change and their access method needs to change too. It is common for a person with a degenerative condition to start using AAC by making direct selections. Later on they may move on to an indirect method.

SUPPORTING
THE AAC USER

INPUT BEFORE OUTPUT

INPUT BEFORE OUTPUT, RECEPTIVE BEFORE EXPRESSIVE

In order for expressive language to develop, we need to build receptive language. We need to know what the words mean before we can use them meaningfully. We need to hear them being spoken in a range of sentences in order to learn their full meaning. We know that in typical language acquisition, receptive language develops ahead of expressive language. This is no different in AAC.

LANGUAGE IMMERSION

When children are learning their first verbal language, they are immersed in it. Children hear it from the time they wake up in the morning to the last thing at night. They are immersed in a language-rich environment.

This is the not the case with AAC. There are not many native AAC speakers. We don't see AAC speakers in our everyday lives. We don't see them in TV programmes or on social media.

There is not a natural opportunity to be immersed in AAC, and so we have to create those experiences.

SELLING IT TO THEM

We have to actively show the AAC user how their AAC system works, and how it might be useful to them. The SLT will need to show the potential AAC user how the AAC solution might work for them. What you show will depend upon the AAC user's needs.

DOI: 10.4324/9781003296850-11

You might model:

- Making a request: 'more bubbles!' or 'I would like an oat milk latte, please.'
- Giving information: 'I can't speak but I understand everything you say.'
- Repairing mistakes: 'something different' or 'I will spell it for you.'
- Asking for help: 'stop now' or 'I am uncomfortable.'
- Telling a story: 'I did something at the weekend.'

The AAC user will not have an SLT on hand throughout their day, and so we have to work with the people who do interact with the AAC user, so that they can keep modelling and creating opportunities for communication.

LEARNING TOGETHER

The AAC user will be learning AAC language at the same time as their carers. We need to openly acknowledge that we are all learning together, and that we will make mistakes. It is ok to make mistakes; it helps us learn.

As the SLT, you can model what to do when you can't find a particular word. Talk through your thought processes as you try to find it. For example 'I'll look in "food and drink", and then I'll go to "fruit". It's not there, but I could say "like orange" and then the person I am talking to might be able to guess. Or I could try to spell it. The person knows it is a type of fruit, so if I just type "m" they might be able to guess it.'

SOME AAC USERS NEED MORE INPUT AND SOME NEED LESS INPUT

Some AAC users will need more input and some will need less input before they get the hang of AAC and use it independently. The following factors are important:

- **Motivation to communicate**: if the AAC user has communicative intent, they will have a hunger for communication.

They will be ready to try AAC. If they are not yet motivated, work on the foundations for communication (see Chapter 6).

- **Attention and listening**: as above. Before we can expect a potential AAC user to follow our agenda, we have to support their attention and listening skills in activities that they choose. Build the foundations for communication (see Chapter 6).

- **Receptive language:** if the AAC user has internal language, they already know the vocabulary and how to combine it into phrases and sentences. They just have to find it on the AAC system. If the AAC user is still learning language or has lost some receptive language, the communication partner will need to provide more modelling, at a level that they understand (see Chapter 5).

- **Expressive language:** if the AAC user has internal language, they may already have an extensive vocabulary and know how to formulate phrases and sentences. In this case, they just need to learn how to operate the AAC system.

- **Cognitive ability**: memory and learning pace will affect how much AAC modelling is needed.

- **Wellness:** if the AAC user has pain, discomfort or fatigue, this will affect their ability to learn. Choose a time when they are most receptive to learn new skills.

- **Sensory impairment**: the AAC system needs to take into account any visual impairment by presenting symbols or text at a suitable size, colour contrast and layout. If the AAC user has a hearing impairment they will need communication partners to be face-to-face, and they will need a way of seeing the language being used.

- **Physical impairment**: the AAC system may be accessed directly with a finger-point or press, or it may require a fist point or press. The AAC user may require partner-assisted scanning, or another alternative access method. They may be learning a new access method alongside learning language and AAC communication.

This is not to say that an AAC user who has cognitive impairment and has sensory or physical impairments will not be able to learn AAC. Far from it. They will just need more input. They will need everyone who interacts with them to be modelling how to use the AAC in a consistent way, so that they can see how they are expected to use it. They will need opportunities to use the AAC throughout the day, little and often.

MULTI-MODAL COMMUNICATION

WHAT IS IT?

We all use a variety of modes of communication: speech, texting, emailing, writing things down, pointing to signs, gesturing and so on. AAC users are no different.

NON-VERBAL COMMUNICATION

Non-verbal communication enhances our spoken communication. Our non-verbal communication is often more spontaneous and more powerful than our words. Communication partners need to keep an eye on AAC users' non-verbal communication, so that they correctly pick up on these signals which may enhance the message.

The following are examples of non-verbal communication:

- Eye-contact: to form connections with people and maintain connection throughout a conversation.
- Eye-pointing: to people, objects or places, in order to reinforce what we are talking about. In AAC, people might eye-point to symbols or text too.
- Pointing: as above. AAC users might extend an arm or use their whole hand or fist to point, if they cannot isolate a finger for pointing.
- Facial expressions: we have a wide range of automatic and voluntary facial expressions to indicate how we are feeling or what message we want to convey about a given topic. This can sometimes say more than our words.

DOI: 10.4324/9781003296850-12

- Body language: we interpret a lot from people's body language. We might gauge how they are feeling, how relaxed or tired they are, or if they are in pain.
- Gestures: there are many conventional gestures that we use to support the spoken word, for example, waving or clapping.
- Vocalisations: we may use noises like 'mmm' or 'uh-huh' to keep the conversation going, or to show our emotional response.
- Tone of voice: we supplement what we say with how we say it, using the volume, speed, stress pattern and emotional tone of our voice to supplement the actual words. This is hard to replicate in AAC, but there may be some phrases where we use italics or capitals in text, or we record a particular message with emphasis or feeling.

Communication is not just about the literal content of a message. The warmth, engagement and sense of connection between the people communicating is just as important as the words and phrases. This is worth stressing at every stage when people are learning how to communicate using AAC.

It is easy to get distracted by the AAC system itself. We need to consciously observe the reactions of the AAC user in order to add richer meaning to the literal message. Facial expression, body language and vocalisations are key to this.

MULTI-MODAL COMMUNICATION

In addition to the non-verbal communication listed above, an AAC user might have several other ways of communicating, which might include:

- Some spoken words and phrases. These might be easier to understand once the communication partner gets to know the AAC user.
- Signs: these are formal hand movements within a sign language like BSL (British Sign Language) or a signing programme which supports the spoken word, like Makaton signs.

- More than one AAC system. For example, they may use a communication book as well as a communication app on an iPad. Or they may use a few signs, plus a communication chart of symbols.
- Writing or typing letters or words to supplement their spoken words. Just writing or typing the first letter in a word can be incredibly helpful if someone has unclear speech.
- Drawing. Many adults who have had a stroke or head injury and can no longer write choose to draw to supplement their communication.
- Using tools or apps which we all use to organise our lives: for example, email, texting, calendar, photos, social media.

Using a variety of modes of communication is known as multi-modal communication or 'total communication'.

By enabling multi-modal communication, we are maximising the chances that communication will be successful. Sometimes, when AAC is introduced, the communication partner gets so anxious about using the AAC that they forget to look at the AAC user and they miss all of the non-verbal communication. They might completely miss the AAC user trying to indicate that they chose the wrong symbol and want to start again. Therefore as part of any AAC training, it is important to emphasise that the connection between the AAC user and the communication partner is of paramount importance. If there is no connection, there is no shared meaning.

AAC DOES NOT STOP A PERSON DEVELOPING SPEECH

With children, families are understandably concerned that introducing AAC might stop the child from learning to speak. Research indicates that the opposite is true.[1]

By encouraging multi-modal communication, including AAC, the child experiences success in communication. This is highly motivating, and reinforces all of their developing communication skills. The use of AAC supports the foundations of communication (see Chapter 6). Attention and listening and receptive language is supported. AAC stimulates vocabulary growth and grammatical awareness. The consistent speech model in voice-output AAC can often support phonological awareness. I have seen clinically time and time again how a child develops clearer speech after AAC is introduced.

This can be applied to adults too. There is nothing more soul-destroying than others not understanding what we are trying to say. If we are consistently not getting our message across, we are likely to either give up, or become distressed or angry. AAC provides a way out of this despair.

DIFFERENT MODES FOR DIFFERENT SITUATIONS

There may be situations where one communication mode is likely to be more successful than another. For example, non-verbal communication is likely to be the most useful in a very noisy environment or where AAC equipment is not available. Communication partners may fall back on partner-assisted auditory scanning or offering choices for the AAC user to say 'yes' or 'no' to. We should value all of these modes of communication: they add to our overall communication competence.

NOTE

1 A research review by Millar, Light and Schlosser concluded that of the 27 cases that provided the best evidence, increases in speech production were observed in 89% (24 of 27 cases). In the remaining 3 cases (11%), there was no change in speech production. None of the 27 cases showed a decrease in speech production as a result of AAC intervention. Millar, D., Light, J. and Schlosser, R. 'The impact of augmentative and alternative communication intervention on the speech production of individuals with developmental disabilities: a research review', *Journal of Speech, Language, and Hearing Research*, 2006, Apr; 49(2):248–64.

MODELLING AAC TO A CHILD

When a child is born into a speaking world, they are immersed in spoken language. They hear words and sentences from the moment they wake up to when they go to bed at night. They are given frequent opportunities to try out words and sentences. They receive feedback and modelling from the adults around them, so that their receptive and expressive language can develop.

When a child needs to use AAC, the adults around them are no more competent in using AAC than the child is. However, the adult can map the AAC onto spoken language in order to help the child learn both receptive spoken language and AAC language simultaneously. This is known in the AAC world as 'aided language stimulation', but I have chosen to use the term 'modelling' AAC instead.

There are several key skills in modelling AAC, which are set out below.

This work lends itself to video interaction therapy, or adult-child interaction therapy. As an SLT you might ask an adult to video themselves communicating with the child. You and the adult watch the video back and comment on good use of the skills below. You can help the adult identify the impact upon the child. For example, 'You waited beautifully, and he looked at you to include you in the moment.'

The adult may choose one or more of the skills below to work on. They might retake a video and you can talk through the improvements to the communication.

It is very important to comment on the positives in the interaction. We all tend to be extremely self-critical and we know when we make mistakes. Your role as an SLT is to be supportive and positive. To avoid overwhelm, suggest that the adult just chooses one strategy to work on at a time. They will go away and work on this at home for 10 minutes per day, perhaps taking a video for next time.

1. BE FACE-TO-FACE

Communication is about connection with another human being. We connect with other human beings primarily through our non-verbal communication: eye-contact, proximity, and mirroring of body language and facial expressions.

As adults, we want to make it as easy as possible for the child to connect with us. We will do this by being at their level physically, so that they can feel our presence and easily glance at us to share their focus of attention with us.

If we are modelling using AAC alongside our spoken language modelling, we need to be positioned so that we can easily access the child's AAC system. We can point to the symbol 'go' as our face lights up and we lean in and say 'ready steady go!'

By being face-to-face, we are making it easy for a child to build the pattern of making eye-contact and then shifting their gaze from their focus of interest, say a toy, to the AAC. We are building their attention and listening skills and their receptive language, at the same time as modelling AAC.

2. FOLLOW WHAT THE CHILD IS INTERESTED IN

Children are more likely to learn language if we talk about what they are most interested in at that particular time. The best way to connect is to tune into what they are doing and then talk about this. When children are learning the foundations of communication, we need to join the child in their world, rather than expecting them to join us in our world. We are the competent communicators, after all.

Once we have tuned into what the child is interested in, we might say what we think they would say, if they could. We can say the words verbally and point to words or symbols in their AAC system. By saying words, we are building their receptive language. By pointing to words or symbols in their AAC system, we are modelling AAC expressive language.

It is helpful to know the child's receptive language level (see Chapter 5), because then we can model language at this level, or just above it. If they understand a few single words, we will model an increasing range of single words. If they understand two words in a phrase, we can model two- to three-word phrases.

It is helpful to give the child a choice of activities so that there is 'buy in' to the activity. If the child is able to choose the activity, they are more likely to be engaged in any interaction.

We might model the use of core words (see Chapter 31), which can be used with any activity: 'more', 'stop', 'you go' and 'I like it' are examples of core words and phrases.

We might also model other words in the child's communication board or in the child's communication book. We can model these words for as long as we have the child's interest: if their interest moves on, we might also need to move on.

3. SHOW THE CHILD WHAT WORDS MEAN

When we say a word, we can point to the corresponding object or symbol, to allow the child to match the meaning.

This is straightforward with nouns: you can point to a cup (or a picture or symbol of a cup) as you say the word 'cup'.

With verbs, you have to catch the action and point to the verb at the same time, e.g. 'you're *pouring*' as you point to the symbol of 'pour'. The same applies to adjectives: you would point to the symbol 'wet' as you say 'oh no! It's all *wet!*'

We naturally highlight the word that is new to a child when we are modelling language. For example we might say 'the bird is *flying.*' We can emphasise the new word by pointing to it in the child's AAC system. We might try repeating it as much as possible. We might look for examples of other things flying: birds, aeroplanes, superheroes . . .

The more abstract a word is, the more we will need to model it in a range of situations. Children with complex disabilities do not have as many natural opportunities to explore the world around them and to connect the meaning of verbs, adjectives and prepositions. We might need to specifically set up some activities so that you can model concepts such as 'wet', 'dirty', 'cold', 'inside', 'on top', 'under' and so on.

4. TALK ABOUT EVERYTHING THAT HAPPENS, THROUGHOUT THE DAY

We want the child to be immersed in spoken and AAC language. So we need to talk about everything that happens, throughout the day, using their AAC system.

Core words can be used in all situations. These include words like 'help' 'want', 'go' and 'stop'. Even with a handful of core words, we can build phrases. For example 'stop now', 'want more', 'no go'. Whilst these phrases are telegraphic, we can model how we say them using spoken language. We would say 'you *want help*' as we point to 'want' and 'help' on the AAC system. We can emphasise the symbolised words as we say them.

Fringe words are those which are specific to a particular activity or situation. For example clothes vocabulary might be helpful when getting dressed. Food vocabulary might be helpful for mealtimes. You can read more about core and fringe words in Chapter 31.

We will probably need to model different AAC modes at different times of the day. We might use a communication board that is laminated and stuck to the bathroom tiles for toileting. We might have a single message VOCA near the front door to say 'let's go!'

Vocabulary will need regularly updating so that it grows with the child. A child might start off with a simple core communication board but may soon need a communication book with a mixture of core and fringe words.

5. RESPOND TO AND EXPAND UPON EVERYTHING THE CHILD DOES

We should assume that the child is being communicative, even if we are not sure.

We should aim to be sensitive to the child's mood, in order to be an empathic communication partner. We can mirror the child's body language and facial expression as we interpret their message. We can use the child's AAC system to model what we think they would say if they could.

There will be times that we are not sure of a child's message. If a child is using one or two words using AAC, it can be difficult to work out their exact meaning. For example, if a child says 'daddy' we may need to check if they want daddy, or if they want to say something about daddy, or if they are asking a question about daddy. We should watch their non-verbal communication carefully, as this will give us important information about whether we have correctly interpreted the message. Non-verbal communication can give us a clue about which communication function they were intending (see more about communication functions in Chapter 35).

6. REPEAT! REPEAT! REPEAT!

A child has to hear a word many times before they fully understand its meaning and can use it correctly. If a child has sensory, motor, language or learning difficulties, they may need even more exposures to the word in meaningful everyday situations. We will need to keep saying the same words and showing the child the word on their AAC system many times before they use it themselves.

We are aiming to make language learning as multi-sensory and embedded in real life as possible. If a child is learning the word 'ball', they will need to see and feel many different examples of 'ball' before they can generalise the meaning. The same applies to verbs, adjectives and prepositions.

It may be helpful to focus on specific words to model each week so that we know we are covering new vocabulary. We might encourage caregivers to explore a new category on an AAC system each week. If we are using AAC throughout the day, little and often, there will be natural opportunities to explore and use new vocabulary. Revision and repetition is helpful, so repeated routines help embed vocabulary.

Early words need lots of repetition. As children learn how to learn words, they may need less repetition of a new word. If we can provide good quality spoken language modelling alongside AAC modelling, we are supporting later expressive AAC language.

Encourage all the adults around the child to keep talking and modelling: it will reap rewards later!

7. ADD TO WHAT THE CHILD SAYS OR DOES

If a child uses their AAC system to say a word, we can add another word. We can aim to use slightly more sophisticated AAC language, so that we are modelling the next steps. If they use a lot of nouns, we can model verbs and adjectives. If they use two-word phrases, we can model longer phrases. If they make a lot of requests, we can model different communication functions, such as commenting, describing, or asking questions.

We will typically model spoken language as we point to words or symbols on the child's AAC system. We might use whole phrases or even sentences when we speak, but we model the AAC system using key-words. For example we might say 'it's *hot* in here', whilst pointing at the symbol for 'hot'. If the child uses their AAC system to say a telegraphic phrase, e.g. 'want more', we can say back the complete utterance, to model correct spoken language, e.g. 'you *want more*!' We are valuing what they said, and at the same time we are modelling the next steps.

8. GIVE THE CHILD TIME TO RESPOND

Children need four times as long as adults to process language. Add sensory, motor, language or learning difficulties to this, and we may need to allow more processing time.

AAC demands more processing time, as the child has to shift their attention from what they are doing, to the AAC system. This requires more conscious effort than just listening to a word.

We will gradually instinctively know how much time we need to leave before expecting a response from the child, but at first leave longer than you think you need to.

The child's turn might be subtle: it might be a glance, a change in breathing pattern, a momentary facial expression or a body movement.

We might cue the child to use their AAC system by moving their AAC system closer and indicating that they can use it. If the child needs it, a verbal prompt might be 'tell me'. Try not to use too much language when prompting a response and avoid prompts like 'use your AAC'. This makes it sound like the AAC is the important thing; the communication attempt is actually the more important thing.

9. COMMENT, DON'T QUESTION

Children tend to say more when an adult makes a comment, rather than asks them a question. Asking a question puts the child under pressure, and we all go silent if there is pressure to talk.

Commenting provides a language model for the child: for example, 'you found a *worm!*' rather than 'what have you found?', or 'you're *dancing!*' rather than 'what are you doing?'

Commenting typically teaches more language than asking a question. The child is provided with new vocabulary. Understanding precedes expression. Many exposures are needed before a child can use a word meaningfully.

10. SHOW THAT YOU VALUE THE AAC SYSTEM

If the adult never uses the child's AAC system, the child gets a clear message that it is not valued.

The child needs to see that the adult is willing to learn. They need to see the adult picking up the AAC system. They need to see curiosity, as the adult explores the vocabulary and combines words to make phrases. They need to see the adult make mistakes because this is how we learn. They need to see the adult use strategies when they can't find the exact word they were looking for. They might describe what they mean using adjectives, or they might say 'it's *like* a bus'. They might try to spell it.

Adults show that they value the AAC system by having it out, where it is easily reached. Adults show that they value the AAC system by taking it with the child whenever the child goes out. Adults show that they value the AAC system by noticing when something needs adding, or fixing, or when the AAC system is missing.

As an SLT, you will probably need to make this clear to the adults supporting a child. Their attitude towards the AAC system will be very obvious to the child. If the adults don't respect the AAC system, the child will not try to use it.

Conversely, if the adult is keen to engage with the AAC, it is likely that the child will be. Siblings and peers are even more useful, so if you can, encourage them to explore it too.

COMMUNICATION PARTNER TRAINING

There are very specific skills which are important for successful communication using AAC skills. Communication partners are key.

AAC is not a natural way of communicating to most people, and so they will inevitably find it weird and awkward at first. The rate of communication is slower, and this can disrupt the normal 'to and fro' rhythm of conversation. However, human beings are very adaptable, and what can seem alien initially can become entirely natural in a short space of time.

There are several key skills for communication partners, which are set out below.

As an SLT you might ask a communication partner to video themselves communicating with the AAC user (with the AAC user's consent). Five minutes is enough. You and the communication partner watch the video back and comment on good use of the skills below. You can help the communication partner identify the impact upon the AAC user. For example, 'You noticed their non-verbal communication, when they held up their hand to say they were not finished.'

The communication partner may choose one or more of the skills below to work on. They might retake a video and you can talk through the improvements to the communication.

The skills below may be summarised in an information leaflet or a communication passport for an AAC user (see more about this in Chapter 30). This might help prepare for a one-off encounter or for communicating with someone new. For example, at a job interview, or starting a new job.

1. USE NON-VERBAL COMMUNICATION, JUST AS YOU WOULD WITH ANYONE ELSE

Communication is about connection with another human being. We connect with other human beings primarily through our non-verbal communication: eye-contact, proximity, and mirroring of body language and facial expressions.

Non-verbal communication is how we convey emotional nuance to our spoken or AAC messages. We modulate the meaning of the message, and hope that we have an attuned communication partner who picks up on these signals. In this way, meaning is co-created. In a good conversation, we feel that the other person 'gets it'. They have interpreted our non-verbal communication to enhance the meaning of the words we are saying.

For example, we might open our eyes wide to indicate the depth of our feeling. We might blink to indicate frustration.

If the AAC user is a wheelchair user, then we may need to position ourselves so that our eyes are at the same level and we can see each other properly. This will help us to connect and read non-verbal communication. This is all the more important if either person has a hearing impairment or visual impairment.

2. CHECK HOW THE AAC USER INDICATES 'YES' AND 'NO'

This is important for checking back a message. If this is the first time you have met this AAC user, it is good to establish the basics.

3. ALLOW TIME FOR THE AAC USER TO COMMUNICATE

Communication is typically slower when using AAC. The rate of AAC speech is generally under 10 words per minute, where spoken language is over 125 words per minute. Communication partners have to get comfortable with silence, whilst they wait for the AAC user to compose a message.

If the interaction is planned, for example a job interview or a health appointment, then the AAC user may choose to receive questions and prepare what they say beforehand. However, there will still need to be extra time for spontaneous interaction.

4. LEARN ANY SKILLS NEEDED TO ALLOW THE AAC USER TO ACCESS THEIR SYSTEM

The AAC user may access their AAC system by pointing, eye-pointing, pressing buttons or parts of a touch-screen, or typing. They may use a head-mouse or eye-gaze to make selections. This is known as 'direct access'.

Sometimes direct access is not possible for a specific AAC user. They may use 'switch-scanning' whereby options on a screen are scanned and then the AAC presses a switch to make a selection. The communication partner will need to wait for longer for the AAC user to compose a message if they use switch scanning.

The AAC user may need a communication partner to read options and then the AAC user indicates 'yes'. This method of access is called 'Partner-Assisted Auditory Scanning' (see Chapter 22).

If the AAC user uses alternative access, then the communication partner may need to occasionally assist. The communication partner will need to check with the AAC user when help is needed. The AAC user may be completely independent in trouble-shooting when things go wrong, and an overly keen helper can turn into a hindrance in getting things back on track.

6. ASSUME COMPETENCE

Our culture has traditionally undervalued people with disabilities. There is still a lot of work to be done in dismantling mistaken assumptions about the abilities of those with a disability. Even the terminology is problematic!

Check that the person can hear and understand you. Ask if there is anything you can do to support communication. And then treat them like any other competent human being.

7. ASK OPEN QUESTIONS

Closed questions are those which only require a short answer. This might be 'yes' or 'no' or a single word or short phrase. Whilst this type of question is useful for clarifying important information, for example at a medical appointment when checking name and date of birth, it is not so useful for conversation.

Open questions or invitations to say more allow the AAC user more freedom and opportunity in a conversation. They expand rather than shut down communication. Examples include: 'tell me about . . .' 'what do you think about . . .?' 'is there anything else?'

8. SHOW THAT YOU VALUE THE AAC SYSTEM

AAC users pick up on attitudes towards their AAC system. Their caregivers or closest family and friends will 'leak' information about their attitude towards the system through their behaviour.

A supportive communication partner will notice if the AAC system is not available. They will notice if it needs charging or a software update. They will notice if it needs wiping. They will notice if it gets accidentally left behind when leaving the house.

As an SLT, you will probably need to make this clear to communication partners. Their attitude towards the AAC system will be very obvious to the AAC user. It takes a very resilient AAC user to persist if those around them are rejecting their communication mode.

AAC
SOLUTIONS

MAKATON SIGNS

WHAT ARE THEY?

Makaton signs are used widely in the UK to support children and adults with learning and communication difficulties.

Makaton signs are taken from British Sign Language (or the relevant local sign language) and mapped onto spoken English. Makaton is not a language in itself, like British Sign Language (BSL) is. BSL is an independent language, with its own vocabulary and grammar, and is as different from English as Arabic or Mandarin.

Makaton is a language programme to support receptive and expressive language. We always speak at the same time as we use Makaton signs. We sign the key-words in the sentence to highlight the most salient parts. For example, we would sign the key-words shown in italics in the following sentences: 'Do you *want* a *drink*?' 'We're *going home*.'

Because Makaton is a visual support, we can model slightly more complex sentences than the person would understand if we were not signing. For example, if they understand one information-carrying word for speech alone, we can model two key-words with signing, because there is visual support through signs.

HOW DO THEY HELP?

Makaton signs help people with communication difficulties by:

- Slowing down the speaker
- Highlighting the key-words in the sentence
- Making language more visual

DOI: 10.4324/9781003296850-16

Makaton signs support all aspects of communication and language. Using Makaton signs often encourages a person to look at the speaker, which helps them give their full attention to what is being said. The signs give visual clues about the meaning of the message, thus supporting receptive language. Makaton signs are an alternative means of building expressive language for a person who has no speech. They also help to cue the communication partner in, helping them understand a person who has unclear speech.

This can significantly reduce frustration for both communication partners, building confidence and social communication skills.

WHO DO THEY HELP?

- Children with developmental delay or speech, language or communication difficulties.
- Children and adults with learning disabilities.
- Children with speech disorders who will benefit from the temporary use of Makaton signs whilst their speech sounds are developing.
- Children and adults who have reasonably good fine motor skills. They do not have to get exact hand-shapes and movements, but the communication partner will support them by modelling accurate signs.

Makaton does not impede the development of speech. On the contrary, it supports the foundation skills for communication, including attention and listening, leading to gains in receptive and expressive language.

CORE AND FRINGE VOCABULARY

The Makaton core vocabulary contains over 450 concepts and is divided into stages for teaching purposes. In each stage there is a mixture of nouns, verbs, adjectives, prepositions, pronouns and function words. The core vocabulary is designed to be as functional as possible with words related to everyday life, such as people, places, food, equipment, actions, describing words and emotions. From stage 1, signs can be combined into short phrases. This allows for a range of communication functions, including greetings, making requests, refusing, giving instructions, asking and answering questions, describing, telling stories, giving opinions, and talking about feelings.

There is also an extensive resource vocabulary, which goes beyond core words. Books and resources can be purchased which contain additional vocabulary for such topics as 'Animals, Transport and Vehicles', 'Work and Education', 'Public Services' and 'Sex Education'. Basic training in the core vocabulary is needed first, so that you can learn how to interpret the line drawings of signs.

WHERE NEXT?

Makaton signs are a life-long AAC resource. AAC users often use Makaton signs alongside other AAC solutions because they are quick and easy and do not require any physical resources.

In addition to manual signs, Makaton has a corresponding vocabulary of symbols. These can be used in visual supports. For example, to label the environment, to offer choices, for visual timetables, written reminders, lists or instructions.

In practice, Makaton symbols are not widely used, as they have been somewhat overtaken by other symbol sets (see Chapter 16). It is perfectly possible, and advisable, to support the same individual with both Makaton signs and symbolised resources. Think multi-modal (see Chapter 10).

TRAINING

It is important to attend a certified Makaton course, in order to learn correct signing skills. Each course provides the opportunity for practice, including using signs in phrases and sentences. Course participants will practise using facial expressions to reinforce the meaning of messages and varying the size, placement and orientation of signs to make them most appropriate to a given situation.

SLTs may train as Makaton tutors, or may signpost parents, carers and school or social care staff towards Makaton training. Information about training can be found on the Makaton website.

RECOMMENDED RESOURCES

There are lots of online resources relating to Makaton signs and symbols. The BBC have a children's series, *Something Special*, which features Makaton in a fun and functional way for young children. Makaton have downloadable printouts of sign and symbol resources on their website.

CASE STUDY: FRANKIE'S SIGNS

Frankie is an adult who has Down Syndrome. He works at his local supermarket, and also enjoys activities like gardening.

Frankie has a few words, but they are very unclear to unfamiliar communication partners. He also uses Makaton signs. He knows over 200 signs and can combine them to make two-word phrases.

Frankie's key-worker arranged for a Makaton tutor to give some basic training to his workplace and gardening group. The supermarket signed up to be accredited as 'Makaton Friendly'. This meant that staff knew how to support a person with communication difficulties, not just Frankie. The supermarket staff really enjoyed the training session and continued to learn signs long after the training session by asking Frankie the Makaton sign for a particular concept. They found this really helpful when signing to one another across the supermarket aisles.

Customers also seemed to see Frankie differently because they could see him conversing with his colleagues.

OBJECTS OF REFERENCE

WHAT ARE THEY?

Objects of reference are tangible, tactile objects which are used to represent a person, activity or event. An object of reference is used to help a person understand what is happening at a given time. They can also be used by the person to request that activity.

Objects of reference can be held in the hand, and can be kept in a bag or on a key chain so that they can be moved around with a person.

An object of reference may be a whole object, or part of an object that is used in a specific activity. Objects of reference will be individualised so that they are meaningful to the person. The object of reference will incorporate what that person would typically see, feel, hear or smell in that activity. For example, an object of reference for 'getting on the bus' might be a safety belt buckle, because the person is used to touching this. An object of reference for swimming might be a section of swimming costume. Scents can be incorporated into an object of reference, so the swimming costume may carry the smell of the chlorine from the pool.

The object of reference is never used functionally in the activity: it is a symbol for the activity. If a drinking cup is used as an object of reference, it will not be the same cup as the one that the drink is poured into.

Occasionally miniatures are used as objects of reference, but this is not ideal. Miniatures do not often feel anything like the actual object, and multiple miniatures as objects of reference are likely to feel very much like one another.

Occasionally, a highly abstract object of reference may be used. For example, the object of reference for 'we have finished' might be a small rubber ring. This is because the concept is abstract and has no consistent sensory associations.

HOW DO THEY HELP?

Objects of reference make words more meaningful for children or adults who are at an early stage in understanding the world around them. They help them to build a predictable pattern of what is going to happen. They offer the potential for a person to reject or accept an activity and express feelings about it.

All those who interact with the person using objects of reference must present them consistently, using exactly the same language. For example, the piece of swimming costume is presented as we say 'swimming'. This will help the person to build predicable patterns: when I touch this object, then this happens. The same consistent language will help a person who has the potential to learn that words carry meaning.

WHO DO THEY HELP?

- Children and adults with developmental delay, learning disabilities or profound multiple learning disabilities (PMLD) who do not yet understand photos, signs or symbols.
- Children and adults at an early stage of communication, who are learning to make simple requests for activities.
- Children and adults who have multiple sensory impairments, including visual impairment and have not learnt spoken language yet.

If a person can understand photos, signs or symbols, then objects of reference are not suitable. Because they are actual objects, we can only offer a limited vocabulary, and it is not possible to combine concepts to make phrases and sentences.

VOCABULARY SELECTION

You will need to work collaboratively with those people who most often communicate with the person. You may agree to introduce three to five objects of reference initially. These will be the most motivating, functional or favourite activities, events or people. You can then add additional concepts at a rate that suits the person. Objects of reference may be stored in a drawstring bag, or on a key-ring, or on hooks in the place where they activity happens.

The vocabulary is inevitably limited, and will predominantly be noun-based. It is possible to introduce objects of reference for verbs, adjectives or greetings.

WHERE NEXT?

Objects of reference can only offer a limited vocabulary, because of their size, and because they need to feel, sound or smell distinct from one another. If an AAC user needs a larger vocabulary, then you may regularly review whether 'on the body' signing or high-contrast symbols are accessible for this AAC user.

CASE STUDY: SAMI'S OBJECTS OF REFERENCE

Sami has profound multiple learning disabilities, including visual and hearing impairments. Sami gets distressed by some activities including tooth-brushing. His care team are unsure if he understands the daily routine, and are not sure what activities he enjoys the most.

In collaboration with his SLT, Sami's care team introduced four objects of reference. These were: a seatbelt buckle to represent the taxi he uses to get to his day centre, a wooden spoon to represent the cookery session he does at the day centre, a piece of swimming shorts to represent hydrotherapy, and a toothbrush to represent tooth-brushing. These were felt to be very different from one another from a tactile perspective, and also were felt to be the most important functionally for Sami.

After two weeks, the team around Sami observed that Sami seemed calmer about tooth-brushing. They reflected that maybe using objects of reference had slowed the staff down so that they spent more time preparing Sami for what was to come. Sami was visibly excited by the taxi and swimming objects of reference. He was less excited by the cookery one. His residential staff fed this back to the day centre and they reflected that the session was perhaps a little chaotic and not meaningful for Sami. They changed the regular activity to horse-riding instead, choosing a length of rein as the object of reference.

Further objects of reference were added so that he had a drawstring bag with ten objects of reference to indicate key parts of his day.

INTRODUCING SYMBOLS
FOR CHOICE-MAKING

WHAT IS IT?

This is a way to introduce the concept that symbols carry meaning. It is a good place to start for a young child, or a person with pre-intentional communication.

The person is offered a choice of two symbols, for example 'bubbles' and 'ball'. The communication partner holds a symbol in each hand and asks 'Do you want *bubbles* or *ball?*' The communication partner highlights each choice with their voice, and shows the person the symbol as they name it. The communication partner observes the person's non-verbal communication. At any sign of preference, for example if the person looks at one of the symbols for longer, or reaches for it, the communication partner interprets this as a choice and says 'You want bubbles.' They would then blow bubbles to make the link between the symbol and the bubbles.

There are countless opportunities for choice-making through the day, but it is helpful to start with rewarding and motivating choices.

If the person does not understand symbols, but does understand photos, you may use photos. Symbols are preferable long-term, because they introduce a more abstract level of symbolisation. A person may need repeated exposures, but may have a capacity to understand symbols. As with everything AAC, a certain amount of 'trial and error' is needed. Try symbols for a while. If the person is showing no understanding of them and is getting frustrated or showing disinterest, then go back to photos or pictures.

We start with choice-making because there is a natural consequence to a communication attempt. It is a concrete way of showing that a symbol carries meaning.

You might start with a choice between two desirable options. This is a 'no fail' choice. Soon you might introduce a non-desirable option, like a sock or a spoon. This will help the person connect the meaning of the different symbols. When they choose the sock, it has a very different result to the bubbles. This will also help to encourage a clear signal for choice-making, be it a look, a reach, a point or a vocalisation.

HOW DOES IT HELP?

- It introduces symbolisation as a concept: that the symbol represents an object, person or activity.
- It gives a sense of agency, and success in communication, where verbal communication may have failed.

WHO DOES IT HELP?

- Children and adults with developmental delay, learning disabilities or communication difficulties who have the capacity to understand symbols, but who do not yet understand a wide range of symbols.
- Children and adults at an early stage of communication, who are learning to make simple requests for activities.
- Children and adults with profound and multiple learning disabilities (PMLD) but who can visually access a symbol.

VOCABULARY SELECTION

Choose vocabulary items that are most meaningful and functional for the person. For example, a child who loves cars and trains might like to have symbol choices for transport toys. An adult who loves listening to music might have symbols relating to music choices.

Start with nouns because these are the most concrete, tangible concepts. However choice-making can also be used with verbs or activities, for example: 'dancing' or 'singing'. The core words of 'stop' and 'more' can be useful, for example with an activity like blowing bubbles, playing music or giving food or drink. Choosing a person to carry out an activity or receive a treat is also fun, for example: 'Mum' or 'Mohammed'.

WHERE NEXT?

If a person can easily understand symbols after a few trials, then you will want to move them on to using a communication board or communication book quickly (see Chapters 17 and 18). This will give them access to a wider range of symbols, the potential to build phrases, and express a wider range of communication functions, beyond simple requesting.

CASE STUDY: BILLY'S CHOICES

Billy is a three-year-old boy with Down Syndrome. He uses about 40 different Makaton signs and understands more.

Whilst Billy's receptive language is very much supported by Makaton signs, it was felt that he would also benefit from some symbols. As we always want to aim for literacy, symbols are a way to introduce the concept that words can be represented on paper. We can then gradually replace the symbol with the written word.

Billy's parents thought that a great place to start would be at the playground. The SLT emailed symbols for 'more' and 'stop', along with a short video showing how to present these for choice-making.

Billy's parents took these to the playground. After a short turn at being pushed on the swing, they offered Billy the choice of 'more' or 'stop', holding one symbol in each hand, and saying the options as they showed the symbol. At first, Billy reached for either symbol, and did not appear to attribute meaning to them. However, after a few repetitions, and with his parents not pushing the swing when he chose 'stop', Billy consistently requested 'more'.

Billy's parents moved around the playground, using the signs for choice-making with the slide, roundabout and see-saw.

Soon Billy's parents were offering these signs when they read stories, sang songs and played with bubbles or bricks. Billy was soon ready for other choices. Because he had got the hang of symbols carrying meaning so quickly, a communication board of 12 symbolised concepts was introduced within a couple of months. Billy had not needed single symbols for long, but it was a great way to get started.

SYMBOL SETS

WHAT ARE SYMBOL SETS?

Symbols are simply drawn images which represent language concepts. They are designed to have just enough detail to show the essential features of a word, but not so detailed that they can't be generalised. Certain design rules apply for categories of words. For example, all concepts representing people show a stick figure, whilst all buildings are encapsulated by a building with a roof.

Symbol sets are commercially available sets of symbols to represent an extensive vocabulary. They are used in symbol-making software and in communication apps. They are regularly updated to add new concepts which have entered the vocabulary.

It is good practice to select a symbol set for an AAC user that will also be used in the environments they access, like education or social care settings. It is also good practice to stick with the same symbol set, so that all AAC solutions for that AAC user use the same symbol set. For example, the AAC user has a paper-based communication book and a tablet-based communication aid, and both feature WLS. Any additional visual supports for that person will also use WLS.

WIDGIT LITERACY SYMBOLS (WLS)

WLS are used widely in UK schools, for general visual supports and for individualised AAC resources. They are produced by Widgit UK. There are currently 20,000 concepts in the WLS symbol set. WLS can be represented in black and white or in colour. They show a variety of skin tones, and in a 2021 update

DOI: 10.4324/9781003296850-19

to the symbol set, gender identifications were removed from the stick figures. Paper-based WLS resources can be made using Widgit's software InPrint3 or Widgit Online.

PICTURE COMMUNICATION SYMBOLS (PCS)

Whilst they were developed in the US, PCS are also used widely in the UK for visual supports and AAC resources. Four symbols sets are currently available: PCS 'original', PCS 'thinline', PCS 'high-contrast' (for AAC users with Visual Impairment) and PCS 'In Context' (for AAC users who need specific contextual information). There are currently 45, 000 concepts represented. PCS can be represented in black and white or in colour. They show a variety of skin tones. Paper-based PCS resources can be made using Boardmaker software, available from Tobii Dynavox.

SYMBOLSTIX

Symbolstix were developed in the US and then adapted for the UK. They were originally used in the Proloquo2Go communication app, but now feature in other communication apps and AAC symbol-making softwares. There are currently 23, 000 concepts represented. Symbolstix are in colour. The stick figures have a range of skin tones and no specific gender. Paper-based Symbolstix resources can be made using Matrix Maker Plus, available in the UK from Inclusive Technology.

COMMUNICATION BOARDS

WHAT ARE THEY?

Communication boards are a paper-based AAC solution, showing a grid of symbols or text. They show the most useful and functional words or phrases for the person who uses the communication board. The grid of symbols may be as simple as four symbols, but it is more common to have between 12 and 40 symbols. The symbols will usually be laid out to replicate typical word order in a sentence, with pronouns on the left, followed by verbs, followed by adjectives and prepositions towards the right of the page.

Ideally the communication board will contain 'core' words: the high-frequency words which make up 80% of what we

like	want	get	make	good	more
not	go	look	turn	help	different
I	he	open	do	put	same
you	she	that	up	all	some
it	here	in	on	can	finished
where	what	why	who	when	stop

Figure 17.1 Core communication board. Widgit Symbols © Widgit Software 2002–2022 www.widgit.com

DOI: 10.4324/9781003296850-20

say. They include pronouns like 'I' and 'you', common verbs like 'want' and 'go', and small grammatical words like 'it' and 'there'. The communication board may also contain some 'fringe' words which are personally relevant to the AAC user. For example a favourite activity, person, pet or place. See Chapter 31 for more information on core and fringe vocabulary.

The words and phrases might be represented by symbols or text, depending on the literacy levels of the AAC user. Children who are developing literacy may begin with symbols and text, but progress to text alone. Or they may just have text alone from the start. Core words are also the high frequency words that children have to learn as sight words when they are learning to read. It can be unhelpful to have a symbol distracting the child from the word shape that they need to learn for literacy, and so there is a strong argument for not symbolising these words.

The communication board may have ready-made phrases, like 'I am thirsty' or 'How are you?', or the AAC user may be able to combine single words or symbols to make novel phrases, such as 'want more' or 'stop now'. For a child or young person with growing language skills, it is beneficial to provide this potential for creating novel utterances.

Communication boards can be made for specific activities. This is especially useful for children and young people. It is recommended that there is consistent placement of core words if these are included, so that the AAC user does not have to actively look for these words (see below: 'A consistent layout').

The AAC user will typically finger-point to symbols on a communication board. If they are unable to finger-point, the symbols or text might be spaced further apart to allow a fist-point. Eye-pointing or partner-assisted scanning are other access methods (see Chapters 22 and 23).

HOW DO THEY HELP?

If the communication board has sufficient core words, the AAC user can express a range of communication functions, including greeting, requesting, commenting, and asking or answering questions.

Communication boards provide visual support for everyday language. If they contain sufficient core words, the same communication board may be used in a range of situations. For example, phrases such as 'I want go' or 'Where is it' could be used in any situation.

Communication boards may be used alongside other AAC tools. For example the AAC user may have other communication boards or visual supports, such as a menu or calendar, to add fringe words. They may have access to an alphabet chart if they are able to spell other words (see Chapter 21 for more information on alphabet charts).

WHO DO THEY HELP?

- Children with developmental delay or communication difficulties who have the capacity to understand symbols, but who do not yet understand a wide range of symbols.
- Adults who have cognitive or memory impairments as a result of head injury, stroke or degenerative conditions. Communication boards are an excellent first step in learning how to use AAC.
- Children and adults at an early stage of communication, who are learning to make simple requests for activities. Adults can use the communication board to model other communication functions like commenting, describing and asking or answering questions.
- Children and adults with profound and multiple learning disabilities (PMLD) but who can visually access a symbol.

VOCABULARY SELECTION

Don't reinvent the wheel! Core vocabulary has been studied and reported in research papers, and the core words are surprisingly consistent between ages, genders, social, racial and cultural groups. It is recommended that you use resources that have already been developed. See the recommended resources for details.

A CONSISTENT LAYOUT

Think about what happens if you accidentally rearrange the apps on your phone. Or you use a different keyboard. What was automatic and easy suddenly becomes effortful. You have to actively look for the icons or keys.

When we repeatedly press the same buttons for the same reason, we develop automaticity. We have established a 'motor pathway' which frees our cognition up for other things. We want to recruit this in AAC. We want the AAC user to build motor patterns for commonly used phrases or sentence-starters, so that they are not wasting effort that might be used for communication. Symbols or letters are always in the same place. When the AAC user wants to start a sentence with 'I want' or 'you go', they do not have to think about where the words are, they just automatically go there.

Therefore, if you are updating a communication board, or moving from a communication board to a communication book, it is helpful if you arrange core vocabulary in consistent locations so that the AAC user does not have to relearn motor pathways.

WHERE NEXT?

If a person can easily understand symbols after a few trials, then you will want to move them on to using a communication book (see Chapter 18). This will give them access to a wider range of symbols, the potential to build phrases, and express a wider range of communication functions.

RECOMMENDED RESOURCES

Project Core have developed a 'universal core' of 36 core words. Their website has free downloads of communication boards using these 36 core words. There is a range of formats, including partner-assisted scanning and eye-pointing, depending on the AAC user's access method. There are boards using three different symbol sets: PCS, Symbolstix and WLS. These include high-contrast symbols for AAC users with VI.

The ACE Centre have free downloadable communication boards in a variety of layouts and symbol sets. There are also communication boards for specific daily activities and fun activities, like blowing bubbles or reading books. The ACE Centre resources consider motor pathways carefully, and core symbols are placed consistently between different resources.

CASE STUDY: ENNIS'S CORE COMMUNICATION BOARD

Ennis is 13 years old and she is a reluctant communicator. However, she does often repeat a small repertoire of words, including 'mum', 'car' and 'Bob' (the name of her dog). These are often interpreted as requests, but those working with her have noticed that she does not always seem satisfied when they respond to her as if they were requests.

Ennis's SLT suggested that a core communication board was introduced, to see if her communication functions might be extended, and if she might increase her range of words and even start combining words into phrases. A core communication board of 28 core symbols was trialled first.

The adults around Ennis started modelling using the words on her board to comment, ask and answer questions and describe people, objects and activities. For example they might say 'stop. We're finished' whilst pointing to the symbols 'stop; and 'finished'. Other phrases that they modelled were: 'want help', 'look [at] this', 'we play' and 'no more'. They tried to use the core words throughout the day, and naturally this meant that they were modelling a range of communication functions.

Ennis initially seemed disinterested in the communication board, but with the encouragement of the SLT, the teaching team persisted. If Ennis said her commonly used words, the teaching team would repeat it verbally and add a word as they pointed to it on her communication board. For example, if Ennis said 'mum', they might say 'no mum' or 'mum gone' (pointing to 'go'). After two weeks, they noticed that Ennis was looking at the board when they pointed to it.

Ennis surprised everyone the next day when she said 'mum' and then pointed to the symbol 'no'. The teaching assistant checked the message by saying 'mum is not here?' and Ennis nodded. The teaching assistant modelled 'you like mum' and Ennis pointed to the symbol for 'like' herself.

The teaching assistant then named people in class, asking if Ennis 'liked' them (pointing at 'like'), or 'not like' them. Ennis found this very funny, and pointed to either 'like' or 'not' for each person. When she chose 'not' like for her teacher, she gestured for her teacher to come and listen and giggled a lot when the teacher pretended to be upset.

From then on, the teaching team combined the communication board with all classroom activities. They made use of other materials on hand. For example, at snack time, they modelled using core words whilst also pointing to real food and utensils, making phrases like 'want spoon' and 'no more biscuit'. In maths they counted out Numicon pieces to match a number, modelling 'want more' or 'no more'.

By the end of the academic year, Ennis was regularly using 20 different core words on her communication board, and paid attention when teaching staff modelled the other words, and when they modelled two-word phrases.

18

COMMUNICATION BOOKS

WHAT ARE THEY?

Communication books are a paper-based AAC solution, consisting of a book or folder of pages of symbols or text. These are organised into communication topics, like 'people', 'places', 'food' and 'clothes', or communication functions, like 'something's wrong', 'I have a question' or 'my feelings'. There will usually be an alphabet page for spelling words that are not included in the book.

The first page of a communication book is usually a contents page, which gives the names of the other pages in the book. It

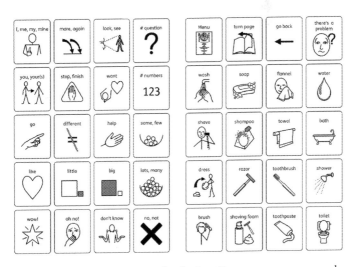

Figure 18.1 Communication book. Ace Centre, acecentre.org.uk.
Widgit Symbols © Widgit Software 2002–2022 www.widgit.com

DOI: 10.4324/9781003296850-21

is helpful if there are 'tabs' on the side of the pages, to help with finding and turning to the desired page. Communication partners may need to model how to turn to other pages of vocabulary in the book, in order to build phrases.

The words and phrases might be represented by symbols or text, depending on the literacy levels of the AAC user.

The communication book will combine both 'core' and 'fringe' words. Core words are the high-frequency words which make up 80% of what we say. They include pronouns like 'I' and 'you', common verbs like 'want' and 'go', and small grammatical words like 'it' and 'there'. Fringe words are specific to a given topic or situation. These will be organised into a relevant page. For example, 'coffee' and 'tea' will be on a 'drinks' page, whilst 'train' and 'aeroplane' will be on a 'transport' page. See Chapter 31 for more information on core and fringe vocabulary.

The communication book may contain ready-made phrases, like 'I am uncomfortable' or 'Please charge my wheelchair battery' or the AAC user may be able to combine single words or symbols to make novel phrases, such as 'you take it' or 'we go now'.

The AAC user will typically finger-point to symbols on a communication book. If they are unable to finger-point, the symbols or text might be spaced further apart to allow a fist-point. Eye-pointing or partner-assisted scanning are other access methods (see Chapters 22 and 23).

HOW DO THEY HELP?

Communication books can provide an extensive vocabulary and means of building phrases and sentences for an AAC user who has little or no speech and who needs support with expressive language. Potentially they can express a range of communication functions, including requesting, commenting, describing, asking or answering questions, telling stories, giving opinions and expressing emotions.

Communication books can also be used by communication partners to model more complex language than the AAC user currently uses.

WHO DO THEY HELP?

- Children with developmental delay or communication difficulties who have the capacity to understand symbols, and who are showing readiness for multiple pages of words or symbols.
- Adults who have cognitive or memory impairments as a result of head injury, stroke, or degenerative conditions. A communication book may be the next step after trying a basic communication board.
- Children and adults who are able to make simple requests and might be able to use other communication functions, like commenting, describing, asking or answering a question, and giving their opinion.
- Children and adults with profound and multiple disabilities (PMLD) who can visually access symbols, and who are ready for more vocabulary than a communication board can offer.

VOCABULARY SELECTION

Don't attempt to reinvent the wheel! There are excellent templates for how to lay out a communication book, using core and fringe words. For example, the ACE Centre communication books detailed below.

The ACE Centre use tried-and-tested vocabulary, arranged into topics which are useful for functional, everyday activities. The topics include: chat, describe, activities, play, spelling, numbers, actions, feelings, shape and colour, position, care, questions and little words.

Of course, you will also want to personalise the vocabulary in addition to the suggested fringe words. For example, a child who is interested in dinosaurs will need a page for dinosaurs. An adult who takes photographs will need a page containing photography terms.

A CONSISTENT LAYOUT

Just like for communication boards, we want to place core words or symbols in consistent locations if they are on multiple pages. This is so that the AAC user can develop a consistent motor pathway for building phrases. No matter what page of the book the AAC user is on, core words which start phrases and sentences like 'I want' or 'you go' are in consistent locations. Core words and symbols which change the meaning of a phrase, words like 'not' or adding a question mark, will also be in consistent locations. This will reduce the effort needed to construct phrases and sentences.

WHERE NEXT?

If a person has been using a communication book successfully but needs more vocabulary than can practically be stored in a symbolised book, then there are a few options.

They might benefit from an alphabet chart in addition to symbols, if they are able to start to spell out a word (see Chapter 21). They might have an alphabet chart within their communication book.

They may benefit from a text-based book, rather than a symbolised book. This is less bulky and easier to change or reproduce, as it can be in a simple 'Word' format. This may be accessed directly by the AAC user, or they may use partner-assisted auditory scanning (see Chapter 22).

Alternatively, the AAC user may be ready to try an AAC app on an iPad (see Chapter 26), or a computer- or tablet-based VOCA (see Chapter 27). This will give them access to a wider range of vocabulary, more grammatical language, and voice output.

WE ALWAYS NEED PAPER-BASED AAC

Even if an AAC user has a communication app on a tablet or computer, there will always be a need for paper-based AAC. Technology fails; phones and tablets need charging, cannot be seen in bright daylight, occasionally they have faults. SLTs will need to encourage AAC users and their communication partners to maintain skills in using a communication book or board.

RECOMMENDED RESOURCES

The ACE Centre has published an essential guide: *Developing and Using a Communication Book*. This has templates for communication books, organised into five stages of language complexity. Each stage has a recommended layout of core words, suggested topic pages, and advice on vocabulary selection. The example shown in this chapter is from a stage 3 communication book.

You will also need software for making symbol resources. Widgit's InPrint 3 or Widgit Online, Boardmaker and Matrix Maker Plus are examples of such software (see Chapter 16). See websites for free trials of the software.

CASE STUDY: GENEK'S COMMUNICATION BOOKS IN ENGLISH AND POLISH

Genek is a seven-year-old boy with learning disabilities. He makes some attempts at speech, but these are very unclear.

Genek's first language is Polish but he attends an English-speaking school. His SLT trialled him with an English core communication board, and within ten minutes he was using this well and even combining two-symbol phrases which had been modelled to him.

The SLT carried out an informal assessment of Genek's receptive language in English and then in Polish, working closely with an interpreter. This revealed that Genek was understanding two information-carrying words consistently in English. In Polish, Genek could understand some instructions containing three information carrying words.

After discussion with Genek's dad and teacher, it was agreed that he would benefit from a communication book. The SLT felt it would be important to have a book in Polish at home, and a book in English for use in school.

The SLT selected a stage 2 ACE Centre communication book, because this would allow adults to model two- and three-word phrases, combining core and fringe words. Polish-speaking adults were to model Polish phrases (using Polish word order) and English-speaking adults were to model English phrases. After a little bit of discussion and head-scratching, it was decided that the layout would be the same for both books. It was hoped that this would help Genek quickly find vocabulary, though he might then make word-order errors between the languages.

Genek's teacher was worried that he would get confused with the different languages, but the SLT felt that we should be offering AAC support in both languages. The SLT hoped that Genek would learn that some adults used English and some adults used Polish.

The two communication books were made, and adults began to model using them. It was decided that Genek's dad would initially focus on the 'care', 'body' and 'clothes' pages. School staff would particularly focus on the 'play', 'food and drink', 'transport' and 'animals' pages.

Very soon, Genek was pointing to symbols, and even began combining two symbols to make phrases. He would do this in both languages, using the word order of the language being used. All the adults supporting Genek were surprised and delighted at how quickly he picked this up.

19

PECS (PICTURE EXCHANGE COMMUNICATION SYSTEM)

WHAT IS IT?

The Picture Exchange Communication System, or PECS, is a highly structured approach for children with Autism Spectrum Disorder (ASD). Before implementing PECS, SLTs are required to attend a training course, as the structure of

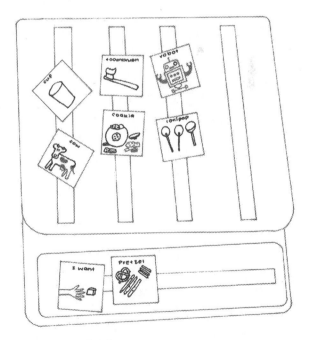

Figure 19.1 PECS book

DOI: 10.4324/9781003296850-22

PECS and the prompts that are used are highly prescriptive. PECS resources, including the pictures, toys and folders, are purchased from PECS.

PECS aims to move children through the following phases:

1. The child makes requests through picture exchange. One picture is on offer, e.g. car. The child has to pick up the picture, initially with an adult physical prompt, and give it to another adult. It is then exchanged for a rewarding object.
2. Distance and persistence. The child has to move across a room to get the picture to exchange.
3. Discriminating between pictures. The child has to select between a non-preferred and preferred picture.
4. Sentence structure. The child builds a sentence constructed with 'I want' + the picture.
5. Answering questions. The child answers the question 'What do you want?'
6. Answering a question 'What do you see/hear?' The possible answers are 'I see a . . .', or 'I hear a . . .'

HOW DOES IT HELP?

PECS is highly structured and uses consistent prompting so that the child learns the exact patterning of each exchange.

PECS provides rewards that are motivating for the individual child. Time is spent to discover what is motivating for each child.

WHO DOES IT HELP?

*   Children with ASD who do not yet have joint-attention or communicative intent and are very 'in their own world'.
*   For these children, it is also worth looking at an approach like Intensive Interaction. Intensive Interaction helps to establish the foundations for AAC communication that we looked at in Chapter 6. An important element in Intensive Interaction which is lacking in PECS is shared joy and

delight in communication itself. PECS is less about connection and more about teaching repeatable communication behaviours.

WHERE NEXT?

PECS is useful for establishing basic requests. However, if a child has the capacity to move beyond this communication function and onto commenting, describing and asking and answering questions, you might want to trial a communication board or even a communication book (see Chapters 17 and 18).

Communication boards and communication books allow greater scope for a wide range of communication functions. Because they are less structured, in terms of both stages and the prompts used, there is more scope for spontaneity in communication. PECS can be difficult to blend with a multi-modal communication approach because the adult is looking for pre-defined behaviours before rewarding the child with the motivating object.

RECOMMENDED RESOURCES

Pyramid Educational Consultants offer PECS training for professionals and parents or carers. They also supply PECS books and toys that are commonly used as reinforcers for children.

CASE STUDY: ELIJAH'S PROGRESSION FROM PECS

Elijah is a six-year-old with ASD. He shows limited interest in engaging with adults or children in his world.

Assessment using PECS resources showed that Elijah was motivated by tactile toys like a squishy ball, a stretchy octopus, a bubble popper toy and a chewy toy.

Elijah's carers attended PECS training (self-funded) and his SLT was already PECS trained. Phase 1 was initiated, using the identified toys and their corresponding

PECS pictures. Elijah's carers repeated the activities several times a day, and he began to request a toy.

Elijah moved steadily through the phases to phase 4. His carers found this demanding, but could see that he was consistently making requests and starting to learn about building a sentence. Elijah was able to construct requests such as 'I want the squishy ball.'

Teaching staff wondered if Elijah might benefit from a communication book, and so this was trialled. It was agreed with his carers that a communication book would give Elijah a little more variety in his vocabulary, and also allowed adults to model a range of communication functions, including commenting and describing, within a variety of activities.

Elijah's carers agreed that PECS had given Elijah a good start in his communication journey, and that now he was ready to use other symbol-based AAC resources.

VISUAL SUPPORTS

WHAT ARE THEY?

Visual supports may be paper-based or screen-based supports which help children and adults to understand language and to help them organise their thoughts and activities.

We all use visual supports. Examples we use every day are clocks, calendars, diaries, lists, notes, recipes, maps, sat-navs and picture-based instructions.

Visual supports can be individualised. We may create a visual timetable showing what a person is doing today. This can incorporate a 'surprise!' symbol for any sudden changes to the routine. We might create a visual task breakdown board to show the steps in a routine, e.g. tooth-brushing or making breakfast.

Visual supports also include behaviour supports for emotional regulation. For example, a 'First and Then' board (sometimes called a 'Now and Next' board), e.g. 'First maths, then computer'. A child may use an 'I am working towards . . .' support, where they collect five stars for class work and then get a reward. Other visual supports might show options for when someone is feeling stressed, e.g. 'I could . . . squeeze my stress ball, take ten breaths, go to the quiet room . . .'

HOW DO THEY HELP?

They provide visual structure for complex or abstract concepts such as representing time or spatial concepts.

They can act as quick reminders of all of the steps in a process if we struggle to sequence multi-step routines.

They help us to structure and regulate our lives. They help us to carry out agreed actions with more independence.

DOI: 10.4324/9781003296850-23

They can help us to regulate our moods and emotions and understand what our options are.

WHO DO THEY HELP?

- Children and adults with learning disabilities or language difficulties who struggle to follow or retain verbal instructions.
- Adults who have memory or sequencing difficulties as the result of dementia or head injury.
- Children and adults who struggle to regulate their mood or behaviour.

WHERE NEXT?

- We might opt to move on from paper-based supports to screen-based supports on a tablet or phone, or vice versa.
- As technology evolves, there are new ways in which people can be supported to live independently. For example, smart devices can prompt a person to carry out an activity.
- Personal preference will come into which visual supports work best for an individual.

RECOMMENDED RESOURCES

Visual supports using symbols can be made using software such as Boardmaker, Widgit Online or InPrint, or Matrix Maker Plus. Templates for making visual supports are often included within the software. Free trials of the software are usually available before you buy.

CASE STUDY: ANNE'S VISUAL SUPPORTS

Anne is a 70-year-old woman with memory difficulties associated with dementia. Anne lives semi-independently.

Her family and GP are worried that she forgets to eat, and as a result has been losing weight.

A visual support was developed to show Anne what food is in the fridge and what meal it is for. She has a different visual support with instructions for heating the food in the microwave and listening for the beep to say it is ready.

Although these supports do not always work, the first two weeks showed that Anne skipped fewer meals. This meant that her weight stabilised and she was able to maintain her independence. Her carers could more easily track what meals she had prepared and consumed.

21

ALPHABET CHARTS

WHAT ARE THEY?

Alphabet charts are a paper-based AAC solution, showing the alphabet, so that the AAC user can spell out words and phrases. They may spell the whole word or start to spell the word. The communication partner may then take educated guesses, much like the prediction software we have when we are typing messages on our phone.

There are a few different possible layouts for the alphabet. We may select an alphabet chart in an ABC format where the letters are in alphabet order. If the AAC user is going to be pointing to the letters and they are used to a computer keyboard, they may prefer a QWERTY layout. If the AAC user cannot point, or doesn't have good vision, then the communication partner may read out the letters and the AAC user will indicate the letter they need. For this access method, a 'frequency' layout is best: the letters appear in order of frequency in spoken English. E, A, R, D and U are in the top row because they appear most frequently in spoken English.

Q	W	E	R	T	Y	U	I	O	P
A	S	D	F	G	H	J	K	L	?
!	Z	X	C	V	B	N	M	,	.
DELETE		SPACE						START AGAIN	

Figure 21.1 Alphabet chart with QWERTY layout. Ace Centre, acecentre.org.uk

DOI: 10.4324/9781003296850-24

A good option for partner-assisted scanning once the AAC user is familiar with the location of letters is to use 'row-column scanning'. The communication partner reads the first letter in each row. If the AAC user needs a letter in that row, they indicate 'yes'. The communication partner will then read each letter in the selected row.

The alphabet may be subdivided into a flip-book with pages showing five or six letters at a time. This can be helpful for AAC users with visual impairment, or those who are overwhelmed with too much visual information at once.

The alphabet can also be used with an eye-pointing communication book or can be used with an E-Tran frame (see Chapter 23). Colour encoded scanning can be used for eye-pointing. Six groups of six letters will be arranged at each corner of the E-Tran frame, plus a top-middle and a bottom-middle location. Each letter in a block will have a different colour. These correspond with six coloured dots at the six locations on the E-Tran frame. The AAC user first looks to the corner where the desired letter is. They then look at the coloured dot that matches their letter choice. This sounds

Space	E	A	R	D	U
T	O	I	L	G	V
N	S	F	Y	X	.
H	C	P	K	J	,
M	B	W	Q	Z	?
Delete letter	Start again				

To use: Ensure you have an agreed signal for "yes" and ideally "no". Hold the chart so it can be seen easily. Speak aloud and / or point to the first item on each row. When the person indicates yes, offer each letter / command / message in turn along that row (including the first option) until they indicate "yes". Speak aloud the letter, command or message they have selected and then restart the process. If you speak aloud something that is incorrect, they can indicate "no" or go on to select 'Delete letter' or 'Start again' on the chart. It is easier to keep track of the conversation if you write down letters as they are selected. If the person is happy for you to predict what word they might be spelling, check you have guessed correctly before moving on to the next word or phrase. Before putting the chart down, always ask if they have more to say. Visit www.acecentre.org.uk for more information.

AceCentre

Figure 21.2 Alphabet chart with frequency layout. Ace Centre, acecentre.org.uk

very complicated, but is remarkably effective once the AAC user and the communication partner learn how it works.

HOW DO THEY HELP?

Alphabet charts provide visual representation of the alphabet for AAC users who can spell but can't write words.

An alphabet chart allows the potential for any new word to be used. This replicates spoken language, which is endlessly creative. A symbol-based or even a text-based communication board or book will never have all the words a person will need, and so supplementing with an alphabet chart gives scope for new words and more independent communication.

Alphabet charts can be combined with other AAC solutions, like a communication board or book.

WHO DO THEY HELP?

- Children and adults with reasonable levels of literacy. Some AAC users may be able to spell whole words. Other AAC users may have 'good enough' literacy: just spelling the first two letters in a word means that an attuned communication partner can make educated guesses at the word.
- Children and adults who have unclear speech. The alphabet chart may just be used with tricky words. If the communication partner knows some context, the AAC user may only need to spell out one or two letters. If they are also attempting to say the word, then the communication partner can use both the first sound and the vowels and intonation pattern that the AAC user is saying. This helps a lot with intelligibility.

WHERE NEXT?

Personal preference will come into which alphabet layout works best for an individual. If one layout or access method is not working, it is worth trying another.

Common phrases might be added to the alphabet chart, as needed by the AAC user. For example, they may need 'I am uncomfortable' or 'Please get my communication book.'

An AAC user may also access screen-based supports on a tablet or phone, or vice versa. They may be able to access a free or paid-for text-to-speech app. Some text-to-speech apps offer different layouts, high-contrast displays and pre-stored messages. See Chapters 26 and 27 for more tablet- and computer-based solutions.

RECOMMENDED RESOURCES

The ACE Centre's website has a range of alphabet charts in ABC, QWERTY and frequency layouts. Some are for finger-pointing, whilst others are for eye-pointing and partner-assisted scanning. Some alphabet charts include core words or useful phrases too.

The Frenchay Alphabet Board, or FAB, is a compact plastic alphabet board. It has finger holes for accurate letter selection. It can be easily wiped clean. There are a choice of layouts, including ABC and QWERTY. It is a small, durable and versatile backup for AAC users who use tablet- or computer-based AAC at other times.

CASE STUDY: IAN'S ALPHABET CHART

Ian had a stroke 18 months ago. He knows what he wants to say, but his speech remains very unclear, particularly for unfamiliar listeners.

Ian uses 'first letter cueing' with his communication partners. He tries to say a word, but if it is not understood by the communication partner, he uses his alphabet chart to spell it.

This improves Ian's communicative success so that he has more confidence when out and about. He also uses this technique at medical appointments. Unfamiliar communication partners used to look to his carers for help when they didn't understand Ian. Now they, and Ian, are confident to persist in working out what he is saying.

22

PARTNER-ASSISTED AUDITORY SCANNING

WHAT IS IT?

Partner-assisted auditory scanning is an access method which can be used with communication boards or books. The communication board or book is text-based and arranged into topics. The AAC user does not have to read the text, because the partner reads it aloud.

The communication partner reads out the possible topics and the AAC user indicates 'yes' to the desired topic. The communication partner then reads out the words or phrases for

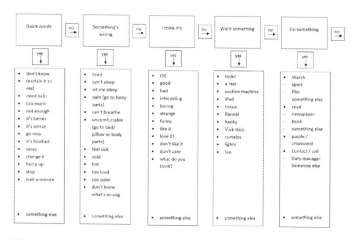

Figure 22.1 Partner-assisted auditory scanning communication board. Ace Centre, acecentre.org.uk

DOI: 10.4324/9781003296850-25

that topic, and the AAC user indicates 'yes' when the desired word or phrase is offered.

HOW DOES IT HELP?

This text-based system provides a lot of vocabulary and phrases in a lightweight and compact format. This makes it extremely portable and accessible in almost any situation. It can be easily changed and modified, with new vocabulary being added at the end of a list.

The option of 'something else' is always at the end of a list of options. This ensures that the AAC user never has to 'make do' with the options available. If nothing else, the communication partner can make educated guesses about what the 'something else' may mean.

Partner-assisted auditory scanning can be combined with other AAC solutions, like an alphabet chart or a computer- or tablet-based AAC solution.

Partner-assisted auditory scanning can be used as a back-up when all other AAC fails. Once this technique has been learnt, the AAC user and communication partner can use it even without the board or book present, because it is quite easy to memorise lists of words.

WHO DOES IT HELP?

- Children and adults who have good receptive language but little or no speech. As long as they have a method of indicating 'yes' (or 'no') they can use this method.
- Children and adults who have visual impairment or who struggle to process information visually.
- Children and adults who have a good working memory and are patient enough to wait for their communication partner to get to the desired option.
- Children and adults who need a lot of vocabulary and phrases, for whom a symbolised book would have to be very large.

- Patients who are receiving end-of-life care may find this solution to be the most appropriate for having their basic wants and needs met. It requires relatively little physical effort (though it does require mental effort).

VOCABULARY SELECTION

The vocabulary can be personalised for the person's communication functions. Their most immediate needs will feature early on in the topics and word lists. There are some very useful ready-made templates available (see the resources section below) which are easily editable.

WHERE NEXT?

Computer and tablet-based AAC solutions may be an alternative. Many of these offer auditory scanning as a means of vocabulary selection. This may increase the independence of the AAC user, so that they are not dependent on a communication partner to read out the options.

RECOMMENDED RESOURCES

The ACE Centre's website has templates for partner-assisted auditory scanning communication books and boards. Because these are in word format, they can be edited for an individual AAC user's needs.

CASE STUDY: ZOE'S PARTNER-ASSISTED AUDITORY SCANNING

Zoe is a 40-year-old who has a rapidly deteriorating degenerative condition. She has retained good receptive language and good working memory.

Zoe has previously used a computer-based AAC solution for her deteriorating speech. However she is finding this increasingly tiring to use. Her vision is affected by her condition, and she is struggling to see text on a screen, even if it is magnified.

The SLT suggested a partner-assisted auditory scanning communication board. At first, Zoe thought that this sounded too slow and onerous. She was used to typing messages, and did not like the idea of needing a communication partner to mediate her communication.

However she was willing to give it a try.

After a week of trialling the board, Zoe reported that it was surprisingly successful. She and her communication partners had quickly learnt the order of options and the list of words in each topic. The vocabulary was arranged so that the most high-frequency messages were positioned early in the options. This meant that Zoe could very quickly request a drink, suction or repositioning.

Zoe requested a few additions and modifications to personalise her communication board.

Over the next three months, Zoe's physical health continued to deteriorate, and in line with the expected progression of her condition, she lost her vision.

Zoe spent her last few days in a hospice. Her family contacted the SLT afterwards to say that Zoe had continued to use her communication board right up to the end. Without it, she would not have been able to communicate essential messages to nursing staff. She used her communication board to say 'I love you' to her family at the end of her life.

EYE-POINTING AND
E-TRAN FRAMES

WHAT ARE THEY?

- A perspex or laminated cardboard frame which has a hole in the middle. It is held up in front of an AAC user who uses eye-pointing, so that the communication partner can easily see their eye-pointing. Depending on the needs of the AAC user, symbols or text will be displayed at the four corners, and possibly centre-top and centre-bottom of the frame. The AAC user eye-points (looks at) the symbol or text that they wish to select.

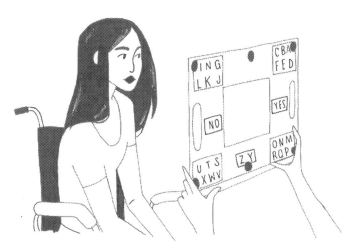

Figure 23.1 E-Tran frame

DOI: 10.4324/9781003296850-26

- Although there are up to six possible locations for eye-pointing, the potential number of symbols or letters can be increased if colour-encoding is added to the system. In colour-encoding, each of the six locations on the frame has a coloured dot allocated to it. In each location there are six symbols or letters. They will each have a colour. The AAC user will first look to the location of the desired letter, for example the bottom right. They will then look to the coloured dot in one of the six locations: this will match the colour allocated to the letter in the bottom right block of letters.
- Eye-pointing communication books are also an option. Each page will be made of sturdy cardboard. Some AAC users who use eye-pointing do not need the hole in the middle, as their eye-pointing is very clear.

HOW DOES IT HELP?

- It provides an alternative access method for people with good eye-pointing skills.
- It does not rely on technology. Eye-gaze technology is difficult to use and expensive to purchase. This solution does not need to be charged and is relatively portable (particularly in an A4 format).

WHO DOES IT HELP?

- Children and adults who have limited physical control for finger- or fist-pointing but have good control of their eye-movements.
- Children and adults who prefer eye-pointing to using Partner-assisted auditory scanning.
- Children and adults who have a good working memory and are able to learn colour- encoding, which increases the amount of vocabulary available.
- Children and adults who have reasonable literacy can use letters and spell out words. This means they have unlimited access to vocabulary.

- Patients who are receiving end-of-life care may find this solution to be the most appropriate for having their basic wants and needs met.

VOCABULARY SELECTION

- The vocabulary can be personalised for the person's communication functions.
- There are some very useful ready-made templates available (see the resources section below) which are also editable.

WHERE NEXT?

- Computer- and tablet-based AAC solutions may be an alternative. The AAC user who can use eye-pointing may be able to use eye-gaze technology. It is recommended that a low-tech AAC method is retained for back-up, as computer and tablet-based AAC solutions need frequent charging, cannot be used in wet areas, and often cannot be used outdoors in bright sunlight.

RECOMMENDED RESOURCES

The ACE Centre has produced an excellent guide for making eye-pointing communication books, called *Look2Talk*. Like the ACE Centre's templates for symbolised communication books, this has templates for five possible stages of language complexity. Each stage has a recommended layout of core words, suggested topic pages, and advice on vocabulary selection.

Liberator stock the E-Tran frame. This is a sturdy perspex frame. Symbols or letters, or blocks of symbols and letters can be stuck onto the frame and removed again, depending on the AAC user's needs.

Symbol-making software like Widgit Online and Matrix Maker Plus have templates for making eye-pointing resources which are colour-encoded.

The ACE Centre also free downloadable templates for colour-encoded alphabet eye-pointing, which can be printed, cut out and used with an E-Tran frame.

CASE STUDY: WILLOW'S EYE-POINTING COMMUNICATION BOOK

Willow is a 24-year-old who has four-limb Cerebral Palsy. They have uncontrolled upper limb movements, but when seated in supportive seating, they are sufficiently stable so that they can control their eye-pointing. They have a very clear nod for 'yes' and head shake for 'no'. Willow also uses facial expressions to supplement their message, adding humour and nuance.

Willow has some literacy and has expressed a strong desire to improve this skill. Willow has employed a tutor to support this learning.

When Willow was assessed by the SLT and OT, they trialled an E-Tran frame with colour-encoding. They started by using four corners and four colours. Willow and the tutor used different resources with the E-Tran frame. Willow learnt upper- and lower-case letters, and a few high-frequency sight words (these are the same as the high-frequency 'core' words we find in spoken language).

Willow soon progressed to six corners and six colours on the E-Tran frame. This allowed the whole alphabet to be displayed at once. Willow's speed increased, along with their communication partners' speed in writing down the letters to spell out the word. Willow made phonemic errors, which familiar communication partners were able to interpret. They would then show Willow the correct spelling.

Willow chose to have a smaller A4 eye-pointing board for when they are out and about.

When Willow employs a new Personal Assistant, they learn how to use the eye-pointing board. A video is made available, and then Willow can support them to develop their skills.

SINGLE MESSAGE VOCAS

Single message VOCAs (Voice Output Communication Aids) are battery-powered button-operated devices which can be used to record a message. The communication partner anticipates the message that may be needed. Text or a symbol may be stuck to the button to show what the message is. This will help build receptive language as well as give expressive language.

There are different sizes and shapes of these devices. The most ubiquitous is the 'Big Mack', which is a sturdy and durable device with a large, round coloured button. It is fairly loud, and so can be used in a busy classroom or day centre. There are also smaller button devices, for example talking tiles, which can be mounted on the wall near a door, or velcroed to a wheelchair tray or table.

An environment may have different single message VOCAs in different places. For example, there may be one by the front door which says 'I'm ready!' and another one in the bathroom which says 'Please help me!'

HOW DO THEY HELP?

Single message VOCAs are a good introduction to voice output. This can be really powerful for children or adults with learning disabilities who have never experienced having a voice.

These devices, if loud enough, get an instant reaction from people. They can be useful for more passive communicators who do not initiate communication yet.

The wide range of single message VOCAs means that we can match a device's features to the needs of the VOCA user.

DOI: 10.4324/9781003296850-27

Some require quite a lot of pressure to activate, whilst some only require a slight amount of pressure.

WHO DO THEY HELP?

- Children and adults who have no voice and so find it difficult to get others' attention or initiate communication.
- Children and adults who have never experienced the power of having a voice.
- Children and adults who do not have the dexterity to access devices which require fine motor control.

BASIC COMMUNICATION FUNCTIONS

A single message VOCA can be helpful to develop the early communication functions of greeting, requesting, sharing a message with multiple people, or adding a repeated refrain to a story or song. The classic first message for a single message VOCA is for it to say 'go!' after an adult starts a fun activity with 'ready steady . . .' This might be used with blowing bubbles, building a brick tower, being pushed on a swing or trike, and so on.

CREATING CONVERSATION

A common problem for AAC users is that communication partners assume they are making requests, when in fact they may be introducing a topic for conversation. These devices can be really useful for developing communication functions beyond simple requesting.

For example:

- Greeting people or introducing yourself. This might give some surprising information, which start a conversation. For example 'I went out with my family yesterday.' It could be a little teaser, to get people interested, rather than giving the full story. This might improve the use of other AAC solutions being used for this AAC user.

- Asking a question to multiple people, e.g. 'What would you like to do today?' For an adult it could be a more profound question, like 'Tell me something about yourself.' The same message can be used to generate many different conversations with different people. This might make a big difference to the AAC user's wellbeing.
- An open invitation to 'Tell me more about this, please.' Often conversations go on around a potential AAC user and they do not have a quick method of indicating their interest, or their capacity to contribute.

WHERE NEXT?

This might be the first step in using a Voice Output Communication Aid (VOCA). If an AAC benefits from a single message VOCA, they may try a multiple message VOCA (see Chapter 25).

Single message VOCAs combine well with other AAC solutions. For example a person with Cerebral Palsy might have a single message VOCA mounted onto their head-rest which says 'I have something to say. Please get my alphabet chart.'

RECOMMENDED RESOURCES

Inclusive Technology sell a wide range of single (and multiple) message VOCAs, including BIG Macks, LITTLE Macks and smooth talkers.

CASE STUDY: HUGH'S SINGLE MESSAGE VOCA

Hugh lives in residential care. Hugh loves to chat to people, but his speech has been getting increasingly slurred and quiet. In a busy day-room people don't always hear his attempts to start a conversation.

Hugh's SLT programmed a single message VOCA with the message 'Tell me about your hobbies.' When the SLT returned the following week, staff reported that

Hugh had been able to have conversation with many different staff members, but also other residents. This simple conversation opener would lead to the conversation partner asking Hugh related questions. Because the conversation had begun, the conversation partner was able to tune into Hugh's quiet speech. Some conversations had even continued over many days, with staff then bringing in a photo or treasured possession to show Hugh.

The SLT provided a list of suggested conversation starters, and each week, a member of staff would record a new phrase onto the single message device. The conversation starters included:

- Tell me about your first job
- Have you ever had a disastrous holiday?
- What is your favourite place on Earth?
- Who would you invite to a dinner party?
- If you could go back in time, where would you go?
- If you didn't do this job, what would you do?
- What are you most proud of?
- Do you have any regrets?
- What do you think about the news today?

It was noted that Hugh's wellbeing had improved with this simple strategy. He had made some connections with residents he had sat next to for months, but they had never talked beyond the 'here and now'. Now they knew a little more about one another, and could reference this in future conversations.

Hugh's family were inspired to make him a memory book of key moments in his life. This could be used in these conversations if Hugh wanted to reference a particular event or role he had held.

25

MULTIPLE MESSAGE VOCAS

WHAT ARE THEY?

Multiple message VOCAs (Voice Output Communication Aids) are battery-powered devices which can be used to record several messages. Sometimes these are completely independent of one another, or they may be programmed to follow a sequence, like the steps in a recipe or instructions for a game. When the AAC user wants to say that message, they press the button.

There are different sizes and shapes of these devices. Some have as few as two messages. Some have four.

Some multiple message VOCAs are arranged in a grid of eight, 16 or 32 messages. These multiple message VOCAs have the capacity to have different 'levels' of messages: they can have different overlays so that up to six different topics might be used. The overlays will display text or symbols to match the message beneath that cell. The overlays can be made using symbol software such as Widgit Online, Boardmaker or Matrix Maker Plus.

Some multiple message VOCAs can be accessed using one or two switches. This is helpful for AAC users who cannot directly activate the button or cell on the device.

HOW DO THEY HELP?

Multiple message VOCAs, like single message VOCAs, are a good introduction to voice output. This can be really powerful for children or adults with learning disabilities who have never experienced having a voice.

The wide range of multiple message VOCAs means that we can match a device's features to the needs of the VOCA user.

DOI: 10.4324/9781003296850-28

Some require quite a lot of pressure to activate, whilst some only require a slight amount of pressure. Visual access is also important: if in doubt, you can request an eye-test or functional vision assessment for a potential AAC user.

The visual display for these VOCAs is static. The only way to change it is to change the paper overlay. This may be beneficial for AAC users who are overwhelmed by rapidly changing visual displays on a tablet or computer screen. The static nature of the display allows them to focus.

WHO DO THEY HELP?

- Children and adults who have never experienced the power of having a voice.
- Children and adults who do not have the dexterity to access tablet-based AAC which requires fine motor control.
- Children and adults who can understand that different messages carry different meanings. They can select a message for its purpose.
- Children who need to show how much they know about a taught topic.

A TEACHING TOOL

A multiple message VOCA can be a helpful teaching and assessment tool. It can be used for multiple-choice questions so that a child can show their learning. For example, it might be used in a literacy lesson for the child to say what sound or letter a word starts with. It might be used in maths where a child gives an answer with a number or shape. It could be used for a describing activity where the child decides whether an item is 'big', 'small', 'soft', 'hard', 'wet', 'dry' and so on. It could be used for categorising activities, like sorting items into 'animals', 'transport', 'food' and 'clothes'.

INCLUSION IN SPEAKING TASKS

A multiple message VOCA can be used to include a non-speaking child in an activity like a school play or shared poem or story.

It can be useful in predictable routines where the same questions or answers crop up. For example, during circle time, where we always talk about the days of the week and the weather. The VOCA might even be shared between different children in this activity.

For adults, a multiple message VOCA might be used at medical appointments to prompt medical professionals to involve the AAC user in discussions. For example, a four-message device might be programmed to say 'Tell me my options', 'What are the risks and benefits?', 'I need to think about it' and 'What happens next?'

WHERE NEXT?

This might be the first step in using a Voice Output Communication Aid (VOCA). If an AAC user benefits from a multiple message VOCA, they may go on to try a tablet- or computer-based VOCA.

RECOMMENDED RESOURCES

Inclusive Technology sell a wide range of multiple message VOCAs, including Super Talkers and the Go Talk range. If you are looking for a versatile device which may be used with multiple AAC users over its lifetime, including switch users, investing in a couple of these devices is well worth it.

CASE STUDY: TATE'S MULTIPLE MESSAGE VOCA

Tate is a lively child who has uncontrolled movements due to his Cerebral Palsy. Tate's family wanted him to use a communication app on an iPad, but this proved too hard for Tate, because he would accidentally activate different parts of the screen, activating symbols he didn't actually want. He was also at risk for accidentally breaking the device because he sometimes used a lot of pressure, and the iPad would fall off the table.

The SLT in Tate's school trialled a Go Talk 9 device. This had three core words plus six fringe words per overlay, and a potential for five levels (and overlays). The core words chosen were: 'more', 'stop' and 'want'. Overlays were created for the following activities: Simon Says, Playground, Reading a Book, Getting Dressed and Snack Time.

Tate loved exploring the recorded messages on the device. School staff set up activities to match the overlays. They modelled single words, and also a few two-word phrases, like 'more dance', 'want swing' and 'stop sing'. Tate especially loved the word 'stop'. He found it very funny when playing 'Simon Says' to first tell someone to jump, hop, dance or sing, and then to say 'stop!'

Although Tate's parents were initially sceptical (they thought that the device looked outdated, bulky and cumbersome), they saw that Tate loved to use it in school. It was agreed that they would be able to use it at home too. This meant that Tate could build his communication skills during the summer holidays.

Tate's parents were so impressed by the device that they decided to purchase one for using at home. Tate had different overlay activities on this, made by the SLT, but the three core words remained the same.

26

AAC APPS

AAC apps have been developed for use with mobile devices and tablets. They may be photo-, picture-, symbol- or text-based. They have voice output using synthesised speech, and there is sometimes an option for recording speech for very personal messages. Most offer different options for the voice. This is important: our voice represents our identity, and so the AAC user has to be able to choose a voice they like.

Well-designed symbol-based apps will use a standard symbol set, like WLS, PCS or Symbolstix (see Chapter 16 for more on these). The vocabulary will be organised into topics or communication functions, so that it can be found easily. There will be core and fringe vocabulary so that the AAC user has the potential to combine these to make novel phrases and sentences. There will be consistent placement of symbols that are repeated on multiple pages, so that the AAC user does not have to consciously search for them. The app will be editable, so that the vocabulary can be personalised for the AAC user. For example, they may add names of family, friends and pets, and have personalised quick messages to introduce themselves or make common requests in shops or cafes. A symbol-based app will also have an onscreen keyboard to allow the AAC user to attempt to spell novel words. This will also offer onscreen prediction.

Well-designed text-based apps, or 'text-to-speech' apps will have a clear visual display of the alphabet. There will be options for an ABC, QWERTY or frequency layout. There may be an option for a 'two-hit' keyboard whereby the keyboard is split across two or more screens. This is helpful for those

 DOI: 10.4324/9781003296850-29

with visual processing or motor impairments, who need bigger cells and fewer cells per page. There should also be the option for prediction. This potentially reduced key-presses, as the AAC user may only need to type the first two letters of a word and then select one of the prediction suggestions. Prediction usually speeds up communication using text-to-speech, and reduces fatigue. The exception is where the AAC user has very good literacy and a fast typing speed. A good text-to-speech app will also have the capacity to store pre-made phrases, possibly organised into topics.

Some AAC apps allow different layouts so that the number of cells per page can be matched to the AAC user's visual perception and physical accuracy. Some will allow personalisation of colour contrasts and distance between cells.

HOW DO THEY HELP?

AAC apps mean that a mainstream device can become a VOCA. This reduces the cost of a computer- or tablet-based AAC solution. It also offers a lightweight and portable device. Screen protectors and cases with a carry handle, strap and stand will furthermore enhance the device's robustness and portability. An angled stand is recommended to prevent posture problems. Sometimes a Bluetooth speaker is necessary, because the volume is not especially loud on a tablet.

AAC apps are especially useful for AAC users who can accurately use a touch-screen. The AAC solution does not stand out as particularly unusual, and it is familiar to communication partners, familiar and new.

The disadvantage of a small device is that it may not be suitable for the AAC user's physical access needs, or visual processing needs. Many people assume that smaller is better, but this is not the case if the symbols are so small on the screen that the AAC user cannot see them or accurately select them. Smaller screens generally mean more visual fatigue. If this is the AAC user's main form of communication, they need a device that they can comfortably use for hours each day.

Alternative access methods for communication apps are being developed all the time, with some apps offering head-mouse or eye-tracking options. Like with all alternative access methods, they need to be tried out to see if they are suitable for the individual AAC user.

WHO DO THEY HELP?

- Children and adults who have never experienced the power of having a voice.
- Children and adults who have the dexterity to access small touch-screen devices.
- Children and adults who need an extensive vocabulary which can be combined to create phrases and sentences.
- Children and adults who benefit from either symbol-based or text-based AAC. They will need to retain their paper-based AAC for when the tablet is being charged and for situations where an electronic device cannot be used.

A GOOD AAC SOLUTION RESTS ON A GOOD LANGUAGE AND AAC ASSESSMENT

Make sure that you have a good idea of the AAC user's receptive language levels and AAC needs (see Chapters 5 and 8).

If an AAC user has relatively good receptive language, they will need an extensive vocabulary, as described above.

If receptive language is currently at a 1 information-carrying word level or below, they may not yet be ready for an AAC app with an extensive vocabulary. There are very simple AAC apps which have a small vocabulary, and some are restricted to photos or pictures, rather than symbols. These are designed mainly for basic communication needs, and do not offer extensive language or communication functions. Examples of this kind of app are ChatAble and GoTalk NOW.

An AAC user who understands 2 information-carrying words or above will need an app that allows them to combine symbols to make phrases, and for the communication partner to model these. Look for an app with consistently placed core words to allow this phrase-building. This should also allow a range of communication functions, beyond simple requesting (see Chapter 35).

SYMBOLS OR TEXT? OR BOTH?

Your assessment will also have revealed whether the AAC user is able to make reasonable spelling attempts. They may be able to use a text-to-speech app with no symbols. If they have emerging literacy (they are making reasonable guesses about the first two letters) then a symbol-based package with an onscreen keyboard will further develop their skills. Prediction may be symbolised, but this may detract from their learning word-shapes. Trial-and-error will probably reveal what is best for the individual, and it may change over time. A good AAC app will have options for changing these settings.

WHERE NEXT?

If an AAC app does not meet the AAC user's needs in terms of physical access or visual perception, then they may require a dedicated communication device (see the next chapter).

Sometimes a paper-based AAC solution is more effective and efficient than a screen-based AAC solution. For example, if an AAC user has uncontrolled movements of the upper limbs and head, or they have visual perception difficulties, then a partner-assisted auditory scanning communication book may be more reliable. There is a kudos in having a computer- or tablet-based AAC system, but sometimes 'old school' is the way to go.

RECOMMENDED RESOURCES

iPad apps need to be downloaded from the app store, whilst Android apps are on Google Play. Beware of apps that require 'in-app purchases' for things like voice output or extra vocabulary. Ideally try before you buy. AAC apps that have been used widely and can be adapted for the AAC user's individual needs are detailed below.

- Grid for iPad: this offers a range of symbolised and text-to-speech apps. The symbolised apps were designed with WLS, but some are also available with PCS or Symbolstix. Super Core and Voco Chat are highly recommended as a symbol-based app, and Fast Talker and Alpha Talker are highly recommended text-to-speech apps. All of these packages are easily edited on the device. The symbolised packages have an onscreen keyboard with prediction, with a choice of keyboard layouts. The prediction can be symbolised if needed. The text-based packages have clear visual layout. The packages allow access to email, text-messaging, social media and other applications like smart devices for music. There is a wide choice of voices and an increasing choice of languages.
- TD Snap: this app, available on Apple and Windows devices, offers a range of symbolised, text-based and visual scene display options. The symbolised packages use PCS symbols. There is a range of layouts and vocabulary levels. There are pre-made behavioural supports included within the package. There is a package designed for people with aphasia which allows photos to be uploaded and notes to be added.
- Proloquo2Go: this is perhaps the best known symbolised AAC app. It uses Symbolstix symbols. There is a range of possible layouts and three vocabulary levels. It is easy to edit. There is an onscreen keyboard, but it is not as intuitive to find nor as easy to edit as it might be. There is a separate text-to-speech app called Proloquo4Text, not included in the cost of this app, but of the same high quality. Both apps offer a range of voices and languages.
- Touch Chat: this offers symbolised and text-based versions of the Touch Chat vocabulary package. This is a pragmatic-based vocabulary package, where communication functions are highlighted. For example, pages are titled 'I want', 'I feel' and 'ask question'. The packages are easy to edit, and the layout can be customised. The onscreen keyboard is a

QWERTY layout with prediction. There are text-to-speech options too. These packages also offer access to email, text-messaging and social media. English, Spanish, French, Hebrew and Arabic versions are available.

- Predictable: this is an excellent text-to-speech app available on both apple and android devices. It has a very clear visual layout and is easily customisable so that the user has the option to use personalised pre-stored messages and prediction. This app offers switch-scanning, head-mouse, and eye-tracking access options. The necessary force and duration of presses on the touch screen can also be individualised. This app also offers 'my-own-voice' software to create a personalised voice.

CASE STUDY: DEREK'S TEXT-TO-SPEECH APP

Derek had surgery and radiotherapy for cancer which permanently damaged his oesophagus and larynx. He has no voice as a result.

Derek has no cognitive impairment and is literate. He tried several text-to-speech apps and preferred 'Predictable'. He tried an iPad Mini, but settled on a full-sized iPad because he can see the cells more easily. He chose a voice which reflects his regional Northern accent.

Whilst Derek would much prefer to have his natural voice back, he accepts that this is the next best option. He has customised his app so that he can easily use stored phrases. Derek also makes use of a feature that speaks a 'floor hold' phrase to let new communication partners know that he is typing. This prevents them from interrupting his train of thought.

27

COMPUTER AND TABLET VOCAS

WHAT ARE THEY?

These can either be mainstream tablets and computers which have AAC software loaded onto them, or they might be computers and tablets that are specifically designed to be used as VOCAs.

Mainstream tablets like iPads and the Microsoft Surface Pro can make effective VOCAs. They will need a protective case, ideally with an integral angled stand and a carry handle. A Bluetooth loudspeaker can sometimes be helpful.

The input of an OT, healthcare scientist or clinical scientist will be needed if a mainstream tablet needs to be adapted for specific access needs. For example, if it requires an eye-gaze camera to be mounted onto it, or if it needs mounting onto a wheelchair.

Dedicated communication devices may be based on a mainstream laptop or tablet, but they have then been built into a robust case with loudspeaker. They are usually mountable onto wheelchairs and can be accessed with switches and alternative mice. They may also have a head-mouse or an eye-gaze camera and software built in.

HOW DO THEY HELP?

These are highly bespoke AAC solutions which can be tailored to the specific access needs of the individual.

The dedicated AAC devices are more robust than mainstream tablets and laptops. The stand, carry handle, speaker and access equipment will usually be integral, making the device easier to transport and set up.

 DOI: 10.4324/9781003296850-30

There are a range of sizes of device. An AAC user with visual problems may require a larger screen than a standard tablet. However, a larger screen requires effort to scan across its distance and make accurate selections in all areas of the screen. This is also true for a head-mouse, joystick or rollerball. An OT's input is essential where there are complex access needs.

The suppliers of dedicated AAC devices are often able to help with customising settings so that the device works in the best possible way for an AAC user.

Computer and tablet VOCAs offer access to mainstream computer applications, such as the internet, emails and social media. Some are compatible with environmental controls.

WHO DOES IT HELP?

- Children and adults who cannot access mainstream computers or tablets because of their physical access needs.
- Children and adults who need an extensive vocabulary which can be combined to create phrases and sentences.
- Children and adults who benefit from either symbol-based or text-based AAC. They will need to retain their paper-based AAC for when the tablet is being charged and for situations where an electronic device cannot be used.
- Young people and adults who would benefit from access to environmental controls and other mainstream computer applications, like access to the internet, emails and social media.

A GOOD AAC SOLUTION RESTS ON A GOOD LANGUAGE AND AAC ASSESSMENT

Make sure that you have a good idea of the AAC user's receptive language levels and AAC needs (see Chapter 5).

If an AAC user has relatively good receptive language, they will need an extensive vocabulary, as described above.

If receptive language is currently at a 1 information-carrying word level or below, they may not yet be ready for a dedicated device with an extensive vocabulary. They may first need to use a paper-based AAC solution or an AAC app on a mainstream tablet or computer. Before they can be assessed by NHS specialised services for this kind of VOCA, an AAC user needs to have communicative intent, have a clear discrepancy between their receptive and expressive language, and have the potential to combine words into phrases (see chapter 47). This may take time.

An AAC user who understands 2 information-carrying words or above will need a vocabulary package (either symbol-based or text-based) that allows them to combine words to make phrases, and for the communication partner to model these. The package should allow a range of communication functions, beyond simple requesting (see Chapter 35).

SYMBOLS OR TEXT? OR BOTH?

Your assessment will also have revealed whether the AAC user is able to make reasonable spelling attempts. They may be able to use a text-to-speech vocabulary package with no symbols. If they have emerging literacy (they are making reasonable guesses about the first two letters) then a symbol-based package with an onscreen keyboard will further develop their skills. Prediction may be symbolised, but this may detract from their learning word-shapes. Trial-and-error will probably reveal what is best for the individual, and it may change over time. A good vocabulary package will have options for changing these settings.

WHERE NEXT?

Sometimes a paper-based AAC solution is more effective and efficient than a screen-based AAC solution. An AAC user will always need a paper-based backup, as devices need charging, and occasionally they have technical issues which require them to be sent away.

In end-of-life care, AAC users often use a paper-based solution, as this requires less cognitive and physical effort.

RECOMMENDED RESOURCES

There is a very small number of specialist suppliers of dedicated computer and tablet VOCAs. The same applies to the software for vocabulary packages. All of the suppliers listed below have extensive experience of this market. They will all be able to advise on possible solutions and arrange trials of these. AAC software such as Grid 3, TD Snap and Mind Express can be purchased for use on any Windows-based device.

It is recommended that if they meet the criteria, the AAC user makes use of the NHS England (or other nationally funded service) commissioned specialised AAC assessment service for their geographical location. If the AAC user meets the criteria, the service will offer a specialist assessment of their needs. If the AAC user does not meet the criteria for the specialist AAC assessment service, they can be signposted to charitable organisations for funding, or may be able to buy their own device. See Chapters 47 and 48 for more information.

At the time of writing, the recommended suppliers of VOCAs and software are:

- Smartbox: a UK-based company which supplies a range of AAC devices and 'Grid 3' software for vocabulary packages. The Grid 3 software is arguably the market leader in the UK, being intuitive and easy to use, with high-quality vocabulary packages.
- Jabbla: A European company which supplies a range of AAC devices and 'Mind Express' software for vocabulary packages. They are very strong at providing bespoke solutions for individuals.
- Liberator: a US company which supplies worldwide a range of AAC devices and software for vocabulary packages. Their devices are particularly robust and tend to have a long life.
- Tobii-Dynavox: A European and US merged company which supplies a range of AAC devices and 'TD Snap' software for vocabulary packages. Tobii have long been eye-gaze specialists, and their devices are robust and reliable.

- Abilia: A European company which supplies the ubiquitous text-to-speech device, the lightwriter. This is a dedicated VOCA, rather than a multi-functional computer. Abilia also supply environmental controls equipment.

CASE STUDY: PRIYANKA'S AAC DEVICE

Priyanka is a 20-year-old who would like to attend university to study psychology. Priyanka meets the NHS England criteria for specialised AAC assessment with a regional AAC Centre. An SLT, OT and clinical technologist are involved in her assessment, along with Priyanka and two of her Personal Assistants.

Priyanka needs a robust device which can withstand her accidental uncontrolled movements. The device needs mounting on Priyanka's electric wheelchair.

Priyanka has grown up using a symbolised vocabulary package with an onscreen keyboard. She now feels ready to move to a text-to-speech vocabulary package. She will need to take notes, send emails and access the internet for her studies. She would also like access to social media and music and video on her device.

Priyanka's access method is a joystick, which needs to be mounted onto her wheelchair tray.

The best-fit device is a dedicated VOCA, which is in robust casing and can be mounted on to her wheelchair. The device has mainstream software, along with her specialist AAC software.

Priyanka now feels ready to explore university options. She will access Disabled Students' Allowance and the Disabled Students Support Service of her chosen university to ensure that she has equal access to her chosen path of study.

EYE-GAZE TECHNOLOGY

28

WHAT IS IT?

Eye-gaze is an access method for using a computer. The term 'eye-pointing' is used for paper-based AAC, whilst 'eye-gaze' is used for computer-based AAC. A camera, usually positioned at the bottom of the computer screen, picks up on eye-movements of the AAC user, and this is then translated into movements on screen, much like a standard mouse.

Eye-gaze for computer games, including educational games, is relatively straightforward. This is because many of the games just require the camera to pick up spontaneous eye-movements. This will result in exciting actions on screen: paint might be splatted, or fireworks might go off. Some eye-gaze games build visual skills like being able to fixate on or track a moving target. This may build the skills necessary to use eye-gaze technology for AAC.

Eye-gaze for AAC or for standard computer applications like the internet or emails is incredibly demanding. The AAC user must learn to make very precise conscious eye-movements and fixate on relatively small areas of the screen in order to make a selection. They must be able to access all areas of the screen. Eye movements are naturally very spontaneous, darting from here to there. To use eye-gaze technology, we have to consciously control our eye-movements, and only use them to scan and select cells on a screen. This requires tremendous concentration and sustained energy.

For this reason, when an AAC user is learning to use eye-gaze, it is recommended that they only practise for 15 minutes at a time and slowly build their stamina. Even when they are proficient, eye-gaze users need to take regular screen breaks or risk eye-strain.

If an AAC user requires eye-gaze to access AAC, then the local SLT will need to refer to a specialised AAC assessment service (see Chapter 47). There will need to be a thorough assessment, involving an OT to select the most appropriate eye-gaze camera. Not all eye-gaze cameras work well with all eyes: eye-colour, glasses, medication and eye-conditions can all affect how well the camera picks up eye movements.

HOW DOES IT HELP?

If eye-gaze is a viable access option, it offers direct selection on a computer screen, just as a mouse or head-mouse would. If the eye-gaze user becomes proficient, they can access other applications like the internet, emails, social media and environmental controls.

WHO DOES IT HELP?

- Children and adults who cannot use other 'direct selection' access methods such as a touchscreen or keyboard, a mouse or an alternative mouse like a joystick, rollerball, glidepad or head mouse.
- Children and adults who cannot use switches as an access method.
- Children and adults who use eye-pointing in their paper-based AAC, and so are already adept in some eye movement skills, such as conscious fixation.
- Children and adults who have the visual and cognitive skills to learn the progression of skills necessary for using eye-gaze for AAC.

Eye-gaze technology is sometimes thought to be a panacea for all complex access needs. However, if the AAC user has poor trunk stability and uncontrolled head movements, this will not be the right solution.

VOCABULARY SELECTION

Eye-gaze is an access method which can be used with the AAC software we considered in the previous chapter.

The AAC user will typically require a simpler layout with fewer symbols or text cells on the page, because accurate selections are challenging. A symbol package will therefore have more pages of vocabulary, and possibly use a 'more' button to access the second page in a category. They may require a two-hit keyboard for typing.

WHERE NEXT?

Sometimes a paper-based AAC solution is more effective and efficient than a screen-based AAC solution. An AAC user will always need a paper-based backup, as devices need charging, and occasionally they have technical issues which require them to be sent away.

Some AAC users who trial eye-gaze conclude that it is too tiring, and they choose another access method instead. Switch-scanning, despite it being an indirect selection method, is generally felt to be less fatiguing than eye-gaze. Some AAC users use two different access methods for different times of the day, depending on their fatigue.

RECOMMENDED RESOURCES

The same suppliers listed in the previous chapter supply eye-gaze cameras and dedicated eye-gaze VOCAs. Eye-gaze cameras vary in their ability to work in different light conditions, and with different AAC users. A trial of several cameras or VOCAs is recommended.

CASE STUDY: TYRIQUE'S EYE-GAZE

Tyrique has been using an eye-pointing communication book for two years. He has a Look2Talk book, with Stage 4 vocabulary. He is able to access six areas of the page with his eye-pointing book. He regularly combines a core word with a fringe word. He is working hard on his literacy and knows most of the sounds and letters in the alphabet and can make a good attempt at spelling the first letter in a word.

Tyrique's family were keen for him to try eye-gaze as an access method. He met the criteria for assessment by his regional specialised AAC assessment service.

The OT set Tyrique up with some eye-gaze games initially. He had to try to select items on the screen to build a picture. Tyrique was able to loan a device which was loaded with a range of eye-gaze games. His family completed sheets which asked questions about his accuracy in making selections from all over the screen, fixating for a given period and tracking moving objects in order to activate an action.

Tyrique's family fed back that Tyrique had been able to access these games. They had been diligent in completing the sheets to track his progress.

At the next assessment session, the SLT trialled an AAC symbolised vocabulary package. The cells were relatively large, with 12 cells per page, so that Tyrique could experience success. Tyrique was able to select symbols, and even built a short phrase: 'I like it.' Different pages of the vocabulary package were explored, and Tyrique tried the 'two-hit' keyboard, where the alphabet was displayed over two screens.

It was agreed that Tyrique showed promise for using eye-gaze as an access method. He tried a few different possible solutions with different cameras. He tried both mainstream devices and bespoke VOCAs. It was felt that a mainstream tablet could have an eye-gaze camera mounted onto it, and that this met Tyrique's current needs.

Tyrique continued to use his eye-pointing communication book in situations where it was not possible to use his eye-gaze device. This included when out and about at his favourite farm, and at the seaside.

VOICE-BANKING AND
MESSAGE-BANKING

Voice-banking is the process for creating a personalised synthetic voice, which can then be used with AAC software.

There are increasing choices for ready-made synthetic or digitised voices that are available in AAC software and apps. It is possible to find regional accents and cultural accents. However, the collection can never be complete.

If a person has never had a voice, they may nominate another person to bank their voice. If a person is likely to lose their voice, as a result of surgery or a degenerative condition, they may choose to bank their own voice. A banked voice will not be perfect, but will retain the timbre and accent of the original recording voice. The intonation will not be completely natural: it will have the quality of the voices of digital assistants and sat nav on our smart devices.

Voice-banking technology is developing all the time. At the moment, the voice donor records a few hundred to a few thousand set phrases. This is in order to capture every possible combination of phonemes and vowels in every word or sentence position, taking into consideration varied intonation patterns.

Recent developments in this field have meant that a recording of a vocalisation may be matched and mixed with an already donated voice. This opens up the possibility of an AAC user having their own unique voice, even if they are unable to produce specific words or phonemes.

Message-banking is a simpler process. This involves the AAC user or voice donor recording just a few very personal messages. This recorded speech will be programmed into a VOCA so that the AAC user can select the specific phrases later. The messages might include terms of endearment, favourite family stories, jokes, or sayings.

HOW DOES IT HELP?

Losing our voice can be devastating. Family and friends and the AAC user can feel intense grief for the lost voice. If we can retain the essential quality of that voice, this can be a comfort.

If an AAC user has never had a voice, they may feel strongly that they want a specific accent or register of voice that is not currently offered. This may be an important aspect of expressing their unique identity in their AAC solution.

WHO DOES IT HELP?

- Children and adults who have no natural voice.
- Children and adults who are able to vocalise but cannot accurately produce phonemes.
- Children and adults who at risk of losing their voice, due to surgery or a degenerative condition.

WHERE NEXT?

If a voice cannot be banked, there is an ever-increasing bank of donor voices. The technology is moving on at pace, meaning that existing voices can be further personalised and refined.

RECOMMENDED RESOURCES

The Acapela group offer 'My Own voice' for voice-banking. Other options are available: see AAC supplier websites for more information.

CASE STUDY: ALISTAIR'S VOICE-BANKING

Alistair has been diagnosed with Motor Neurone Disease. He knows that he will, at some stage, lose his voice.

Alistair enjoys quick repartee and is able to amuse his family and friends with a range of funny voices. His children request specific characters who have set phrases.

When Alistair reported to the SLT that people were struggling to hear him on virtual video calls, the SLT knew that it was time to talk about voice-banking. She talked Alistair through the various options.

Alistair had a Scottish accent, and it was not difficult to find a standard voice within AAC software. He felt that he did not have the stamina nor the inclination to bank his voice. However, he was interested in message-banking. He decided to ask his family for the key stories or phrases that they would like him to record onto his VOCA. Alistair added a few special messages for his family that he felt would be important when he could no longer speak.

Alistair and his family found this a very emotional experience, and it was not easy to anticipate the loss of his voice. However, when Alistair did lose his voice, they were all glad that they had a repertoire of his funny voices to draw on in the darkest times. They agreed that laughing and crying together in the last weeks was precipitated by some of the recorded messages, and had helped them to feel close to Alistair at the end of his life.

COMMUNICATION PASSPORTS

30

Communication passports are a quick guide, in the form of a leaflet, card, video or even an app, for supporting a person's communication. In the context of AAC, a communication passport will give information about what AAC the person uses, and what communication partners can do to help.

Ideally, the AAC user will be central in creating the communication passport. The form and the content will be developed with them, so that they feel comfortable in promoting it with their communication partners.

It might include photos of what the AAC looks like, and how it should be set up, for example if an angled rest should be used, and if there is access equipment like a joystick to position correctly.

It might include communication strategies such as 'give me time' and 'check how I indicate "yes" and "no".' For a child, it may include strategies for modelling language using the AAC.

The AAC user may use multiple AAC solutions. For example, they have a communication book and also a VOCA. The communication passport might set out the situations where each of these is most helpful.

Communication passports can include information about the person's likes and dislikes, strengths and needs. This may include their physical and sensory needs, and strategies to support their wellbeing.

The communication passport will need to be reviewed yearly, in case the AAC user's needs change, or their AAC solution changes.

138

DOI: 10.4324/9781003296850-33

HOW DOES IT HELP?

It is a quick reference guide for new communication partners. It may also help to establish consistent support where an AAC user has multiple carers.

A communication passport is especially useful if the AAC user is undertaking a transition. For example, between school and college, or from the family home to a residential care setting.

WHO DOES IT HELP?

- Children and adults who use AAC.
- Communication partners, new and established.

RECOMMENDED RESOURCES

CALL Scotland have some templates for creating communication passports. See communicationpassports.org.uk.

RIX Wiki is an app-based communication passport. There are options for including a diary for appointments, and for communicating remotely with key people.

CASE STUDY: ELISE'S COMMUNICATION PASSPORT

Elise accesses a few different day centres and leisure activities, and occasionally respite care away from her family. This means that she interacts with a wide range of staff and volunteers, who may not see her for weeks at a time.

Elise and her SLT used a template to make an A5 double-sided communication passport. This gave some basic information about Elise, including her likes and dislikes.

It gave a brief guide to how she uses her communication board and alphabet chart, and how she indicates 'yes' and 'no'.

Elise's family and carers always make sure that a copy of the communication passport is sent by email if Elise is starting a new activity. A laminated copy is tucked in her wheelchair and fastened with springy elastic, so that Elise can pull it out when it is needed.

Elise feels that she can prompt staff and volunteers to use her AAC now, where previously it felt very awkward and impossible to explain.

BUILDING
LANGUAGE
SKILLS WITH AAC

31

CORE AND FRINGE VOCABULARY

WHAT ARE THEY?

'Core' words make up approximately 80 per cent of our everyday conversation. They are the small grammatical words including pronouns, general verbs, determiners, conjunctions and prepositions, often described as the 'little' words. They include 'I', 'you', 'we', 'am', 'are', 'is', 'have', 'it', 'the', 'a', 'this', 'that', 'here', 'there', 'and', 'but' and so on.

'Fringe' words are the content words that are specific to a particular topic. They can be nouns, specific verbs, adjectives and adverbs. Fringe words would include 'banana', 'avocado', 'dance', 'relax', 'stretchy', 'recycled' and so on.

WHY ARE CORE WORDS IMPORTANT?

Core words can be combined with fringe words to make sentences. For example '*I want to go to the* cinema' and '*Can you see my* glasses?' (where core words are italicised). Core words will appear in all phrases and sentences, no matter what the topic. This makes them essential for phrase- and sentence-building.

We can also make a lot of useful everyday phrases with core words alone. For example 'go and look', 'put it here', 'I like that'. Some of these will be telegraphic phrases (not grammatically perfect), but this is sometimes necessary, to allow for quick and functional messages. For example 'why you go?', 'I not finished', 'she do it'.

There has been a lot of attention on core words in recent years in the AAC world. This was in response to an over-representation of nouns in AAC systems. This did not allow for functional communication, or the development of grammar.

DOI: 10.4324/9781003296850-35

We are aiming for a balance between core and fringe, with core words being used to start sentences, and to make up the quick, essential messages that we need throughout the day.

HOW DO WE REPRESENT CORE WORDS IN AAC SOLUTIONS?

Core words are abstract and therefore hard to represent with symbols. There is a strong argument that they are so abstract they may as well be represented by the word alone. This is the recommendation for AAC users who are learning literacy: if they have to learn an abstract shape, they may as well learn the whole word for the high-frequency core words. We want them to learn the word-shape of the core word, and a symbol above or below the word can be a distraction.

CONSISTENT LAYOUT OF CORE VOCABULARY

AAC users need easy access to core words. Core words might be placed on the first page of a communication book, possibly in

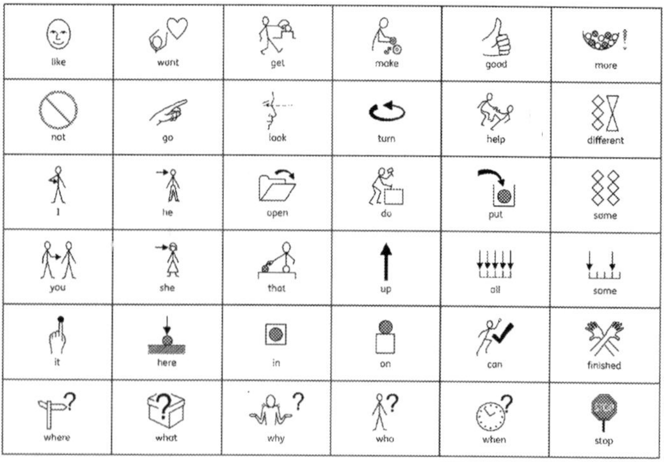

Figure 31.1 Core communication board. Ace Centre, acecentre.org.uk. Widgit Symbols © Widgit Software 2002–2022 www.widgit.com

a fold-out page if the AAC user needs extensive core. Another good solution is to have core words in a consistent place on every page of a communication book or vocabulary package. In the ACE Centre's communication books, core words are consistently placed on the left-hand page of every open page. Core words are on the left, and fringe words are on the right. This reflects the word order of English: core words often start the phrase or sentence.

A consistent layout of core words is important for motor planning. We don't want to think about where our icons are on our phone: we just want to automatically tap them. We want this in AAC solutions too. AAC users don't want to have to look for core words: they just want to automatically select them. If they are always consistently placed, AAC users develop automaticity and can easily locate and use core words.

USING CORE WORDS FOR ALL SITUATIONS

A communication board of just core words can be very useful. For instance, in the core board shown above, we can use phrases like 'I not like it', 'you go now', 'open it', 'put it there', 'who that?' and 'when go?' Whilst these may be telegraphic, they are very functional for quick, everyday messages.

Communication partners will need to model these core words and phrases, to help the AAC user learn their locations. If the AAC user is still learning language, then they will also need to hear these words and phrases in context to learn their meaning. These phrases will need to be repeated a lot, throughout the day (see Chapters 9 and 11). We might systematically target core words, to ensure that they are repeated enough.

Often we have resources in our environment which can be used for fringe words. For example, if choosing a snack or ordering from a menu, we could just use core words and point to what we want (the real object or the items on the menu are the fringe words). This might also work if we were talking about clothes when we are next to our open wardrobe, or if we were talking about music or books when we can point to them.

CORE WORDS PLUS THE ALPHABET

For AAC users who have reasonable literacy, they may be able to manage with a communication board with core words on one side and an alphabet chart on the other. This is also the structure of some apps and vocabulary packages, for example 'Alpha Core' on Grid for iPad.

RECOMMENDED RESOURCES

The ACE Centre have a range of core communication boards as free downloads on their website. Their book *Developing and Using a Communication Book* has templates for communication books, organised into five possible stages of language complexity. Each stage has a recommended layout of core words, suggested topic pages, and advice on vocabulary selection.

Project Core is a highly recommended website which has a wealth of resources around core vocabulary, including a suite of eLearning modules. They have developed a 'universal core' of 36 core words. They have free downloads of communication boards using these 36 core words, in a range of formats, and with three different symbol sets: PCS, Symbolstix and WLS. These include high-contrast symbols for AAC users with VI, and formats that allow partner-assisted scanning or eye-pointing.

PERSONALISING THE VOCABULARY

32

WHY?

What we communicate about is part of our identity. We have a personal vocabulary that is different from every other human being.

The best way to enable a personal vocabulary is to support literacy in AAC solutions. If a person is able to spell, even if it is just the first two letters in a word, they may be able to make use of prediction (either software prediction as part of their AAC app, or human prediction in the form of an attuned communication partner). Being able to spell means that the AAC user potentially has access to any word in the language.

If spelling is not currently an option, then we will need to make sure that the vocabulary in the AAC solution has some personalised vocabulary.

This might include:

- Names of family, friends, pets, colleagues, peers
- Significant places, shops, cafes, holiday destinations
- Favourite TV shows, films, music, games
- Specific equipment including AAC and personal care
- Hobbies, activities and interests
- Special events in their life, past or present
- Favourite food and drink, clothes, make-up
- Words associated with their peer group
- Swear words and words associated with their culture or dialect.

WHEN THE WORD IS NOT THERE

We cannot possibly anticipate every word a person will ever need. The AAC user needs to be able to indicate when this happens so that they can use other strategies. They might even have a page of their book or package devoted to repairing communication breakdowns in this way.

Strategies might include:

- Having an option for 'something else' on each page of vocabulary.
- Spelling the word using an alphabet chart or onscreen keyboard.
- Describing the word by using other words in the AAC system.
- Saying 'it's similar to' or 'it's different from'.
- Signposting to another person or resource, e.g. 'look in my calendar'.

ENABLING THE AAC USER TO UPDATE THEIR VOCABULARY

Whilst the SLT may initially help to personalise the vocabulary, you do not want to be the only person who is able to do this.

It is essential that the AAC user, or a nominated person, can update the vocabulary. A child's vocabulary will change as they become a young person. Someone who starts a new job or activity will need new vocabulary associated with this. The AAC user may feel that some words just don't suit them anymore, and they may want to update them.

It is helpful to have a space at the bottom of each page of a communication book saying 'something else'. This gives a prompt for the communication partner to use the strategies above to guess a word that is not there. It can be useful to have some space to write new words at the bottom of a page, though sometimes we find that the navigation of a book gets complicated when this happens. Often words are duplicated, because the communication partner didn't realise the word was already in the book, but on a different page. A solution might be to keep a running list at the back of the book. The nominated person can check whether these are already in the book and can add them if needed.

The SLT will need to train the AAC user or their nominated person in how to update the vocabulary in a communication book. This will need to include sharing the rationale for how the book is arranged. For example, it may be topic-based, or it may be organised by communication functions.

If the AAC user has vocabulary package on an app or software, then the SLT may demonstrate how to edit the vocabulary. They may then signpost them to training. The AAC apps and vocabulary packages that are recommended in this book have associated training from the relevant suppliers online. If an AAC user has purchased their own AAC device and software, then they will usually be able to access aftercare and support from the supplier.

33

BUILDING VOCABULARY SKILLS

An AAC system will potentially have a lot of vocabulary, perhaps several thousand words. We need a way of organising this vocabulary so that the AAC user can efficiently locate and use words.

There are a few different ways of organising vocabulary.

We can arrange vocabulary into activities, for example 'personal care', or 'going out'. The nouns, verbs, adjectives associated with these activities will be displayed on the relevant page. There may be sentence starters such as 'I need' or 'Can you'. This method of organising vocabulary will duplicate vocabulary, and the same words will be in multiple locations. As much as possible, it is recommended that the same words are located in the same place across multiple pages, though this is extremely challenging.

Alternatively, vocabulary can be arranged into topics or categories, for example 'food and drink', 'transport', 'animals', 'actions', 'describing', and so on. These categories can be further subdivided into sub-categories, so that within 'food and drink' there might be 'fruit', 'vegetables', 'snacks', 'main meals' and so on.

It is helpful if there is also access to 'core' words, so that core words can be easily combined with 'fringe' words in the category pages. For example, *'more* bubbles', 'coffee *no* milk' (the core words are italicised). A good solution is to have a fold-out page of core words at the start of the book, or have a consistent layout of core words on the left side of every page of fringe words (see Chapter 31 for more about core and fringe vocabulary).

DOI: 10.4324/9781003296850-37

Some AAC solutions organise vocabulary into communication functions. For example 'I am asking a question' or 'I am telling you something'. PODD (Pragmatic Organisation Dynamic Display) uses this type of organisation.

I would recommend that you don't reinvent the wheel and use an already invented way of organising vocabulary. The ACE Centre have developed a layout for core and fringe vocabulary in a communication book (see Chapter 18) which is highly recommended. See Chapters 26 and 27 for recommended vocabulary packages for computer- or tablet-based VOCAs.

FAMILIARISATION OF VOCABULARY

We might initially focus upon daily activities. For example, using the clothes page when getting dressed, and using the food and drinks page at mealtimes or when shopping. The AAC user might use their 'people' page to initiate a conversation about specific people, or when looking at photos. They might use the 'transport' and 'places' pages to plan a trip.

VOCABULARY GAMES

'Find something that is . . .' is a fun game to play. It might be 'something that has wheels' or 'wings' or something that's wet or smelly or squishy.

'What goes with . . .' is also fun. 'What goes with ice-cream?' or 'What goes with an elephant?' You can be as silly or as sensible as you like.

We might try specific games or activities to target a page of vocabulary. 'Simon Says' is great for teaching verb locations. The 'describing' page might be used for a feely bag or a guessing game.

For children, Orchard Toys have a brilliant range of games which use everyday vocabulary. For example 'Shopping List', 'Tummy Ache' (food and household items), 'Let's Go' (animals and transport) and 'Where Do I Live?' (animals and places).

There are many ways to generate vocabulary, and you can use your creativity. You might play games like 'I went on holiday and I took . . .' or 'I made a potion and I put in . . .' You might play 'Would you rather . . .' For example, 'Would you rather have a pet elephant or a pet giraffe?', 'Would you rather fly a helicopter or ride on a hot-air balloon?' and so on.

You might use a story-building structure, for example 'There was once a . . .' 'who went to the . . .' 'They had an accident with a . . .' 'They were saved by a . . .'

BOOKS

My favourite book to generate vocabulary is Pippa Goodhart's *You Choose!* With this book, you can help a child to imagine being able to go anywhere, live anywhere, choose clothes, furniture, pets, friends, activities and jobs.

For adults, magazines, books or websites may offer opportunities to explore vocabulary. You might opt to subscribe to a 'photo of the day' or collect a few art, photography or travel magazines. A photo or piece of art might allow you to explore multiple pages of vocabulary, for example parts of the body, clothes, actions, colours and places.

NAVIGATION SKILLS

In order for an AAC user to use their communication book or vocabulary package, they need to have categorisation skills. You might assess this by seeing if they can sort words into categories, for example 'parts of the body' or 'clothes'. Once they have their AAC solution, you can help them practise this skill by giving them words and asking them to find them in their AAC system.

BUILDING PHRASES
AND SENTENCES

WHY?

In order to have true language, we need to combine words into phrases and sentences. Whilst it is possible to have an AAC system where phrases are ready-made, ideally we want AAC users to have the potential to create novel utterances.

STAGES OF LANGUAGE DEVELOPMENT

In typical spoken language development, children go through predictable stages in their expressive language.[1] These are summarised below.

I have not referenced age norms because these stages have not been standardised for an AAC population. The AAC population is diverse, and will likely go through grammatical stages at very different rates. Because AAC users are not immersed in AAC language in the way that speaking children are immersed in spoken language, the rate of acquisition is likely to be slower. The order of acquisition may be affected by the capacity of their AAC solution to reflect these grammatical markers.

AAC language tends to be telegraphic for longer, and there may always be circumstances where quick messages need to be telegraphic. AAC language is more effortful and time-consuming, and so it is efficient to be brief and miss out grammatical morphemes. For example, an AAC user might say 'Stop! medicine' even though they are perfectly capable of saying 'Wait a minute, I haven't had my medicine yet.'

Stage	Description	Examples
Prelinguistic	The child does not yet have communicative intent. They may signal their wants and needs, but are doing this accidentally, and an attuned adult interprets their non-verbal communication.	
Single words	The child starts to say single words. These are usually words that appear frequently in the child's environment.	Daddy, mummy, teddy, cup, car, light, gone, more
	Some phrases are used, but they are whole units, and the separate words don't appear in different combinations	Want-it, get-it, up-you-come
Early combinations (sometimes known as 'telegraphic')	Agent + action Action + object Agent + action + object Object + object, or Agent + Agent Negative + object or action Grammatical morphemes may be used, but as whole units. They are not yet creatively added to words.	Daddy eat Kick ball Mummy read book Ball and book; me and mummy No ball; no sleep Gone

Stage	Description	Examples
Multi-word phrases, including grammatical morphemes	Present progressive verbs (-ing)	Cooking
	Prepositions	Ball in cup
	Auxiliary verbs	Want to eat, have to go
	Contractible copula verbs (they need a verb or adjective)	I am going or I'm hot
	Regular plural	Doggies
	Irregular past tense	Went, fell, broke
	Possessive 's	Mummy's ice cream
	Uncontractible copula (they are not attached to a verb or adjective).	I am. (In response to a question like 'Are you going?')
	Articles 'the' and 'a'	The dog. A cat.
	Regular past tense	I laughed
	Regular third-person present tense	She laughs
	Irregular third-person present tense	She does, she has

THE IMPORTANCE OF MODELLING

Children need to hear spoken language in order to internalise correct word order and grammatical morphemes. This way, even if they can't speak, they can judge whether a phrase or sentence 'sounds right'. This internalised receptive language is the precursor to being able to use correct expressive forms (see also: Chapter 9: 'Input before output' and Chapter 11: 'Modelling AAC to a child').

It is recommended that we use correct sentence structure and grammar as we speak, even if we are modelling key words when we show symbol combinations. For example, we might say 'It's time to go outside now' as we point to the symbols 'go' and 'outside'.

ADD ONE OR TWO WORDS

A useful strategy is to add one or two words to what the child is currently saying, using their AAC. If they are using single words, for example 'dog', then the adult might say 'Yes, the dog's eating' as they point to the symbols 'dog' and 'eat'. If the child has just combined the symbols 'dog' and 'eat', then the adult might add 'Yes, he's eating a biscuit. He likes it' as they point to the symbols 'eat', 'biscuit' and 'like'. The adult has the freedom to choose what to add, depending on the vocabulary available. This is just like in spoken language modelling: it is creative and free, though there will a lot of repetition in order to build receptive language.

STRUCTURED APPROACHES

As an SLT, you may target specific phrase structures. It is possible to use the same resources and activities that you would for a speaking child. For example, 'Simon Says' is an excellent game to target 'Agent + Object' phrases, and this can be played using a communication book or vocabulary package.

If you are using picture-based resources, then make sure that they are accessible for the child, in terms of their visual skills. Make sure that the picture (or video) is visually clear, without too much background detail. Some of the more cartoony resources may not be suitable for a child who has visual impairment or visual processing difficulties. ColorCards offer high-quality images, targeting many different language skills.

Language through Colour and Colourful Semantics can be used with AAC solutions. Don't be tempted to match the colour of the AAC system with the colours of the language programme: this is incredibly time-consuming and ultimately frustrating because in AAC solutions the same word may be used flexibly. However, the sentence structures being targeted in these programmes can inform work with an AAC-using child.

WORD PREDICTION SOFTWARE: THE PROS AND CONS

Word prediction software is sometimes available in AAC apps and vocabulary packages, so that the software anticipates the possible next word. There is a danger that the child will keep selecting the next suggested word without understanding it, and that adults may assume language competence. This is similar to how approaches like *Colourful Semantics* can become a matching game.

It is important that the SLT observe the child when they are constructing a sentence to see if they are selecting the next suggested word automatically, or making more considered choices. Of course, a good language assessment will also be useful here. An informal assessment might involve asking the child if a sentence makes sense or matches a picture.

An alternative approach to building language competence is the SCORE vocabulary.[2] The child learns how to use grammatical morphemes themselves, rather than the software predicting them. Proponents of the SCORE approach argue that the AAC user reaches true linguistic competence because they actively have to process and produce grammatical elements.

TRACKING PROGRESS

Just like in spoken language development, it is useful to transcribe a child's AAC language to analyse the length of their utterances and which sentence structures they are using. Specific objectives may be set around phrase-building. For example, if a child tends to use single words only, the SLT might set an objective for the child to use two-word combinations, e.g. agent + action and action + object. These will be prompted in much the same way as for spoken language. For example, talking through everyday activities, playing games, showing pictures, video clips, acting out, reading books, and so on. For more information on setting objectives, see Chapter 46.

NOTES

1 Adapted from Brown, R., *A First Language: The Early Stages*. Cambridge, MA: Harvard University Press, 1973.
2 See Jabbla UK for more information about the SCORE vocabulary.

COMMUNICATION FUNCTIONS

WHAT ARE THEY?

Communication functions, or language functions, describe why we communicate. They relate to our pragmatic use of language.

There is a tendency when introducing AAC to focus on requesting. This is valid initially: it shows the child the power of communication. There is a consequence to their communication. This can help to establish communicative intent.

We then need to move on to model a range of communicative functions.

There is not a set order of acquisition when it comes to communicative functions. Several communication functions might develop concurrently. However, some functions are more concrete, in that they relate to objects or actions that can be seen and heard in the here-and-now, whilst others are more abstract, in that they relate to events in the past or future, or to thoughts, ideas, opinions and emotions.

If I were to group communication functions into 'early' or 'late', they might look like the table on the following page.

I expect that there will be huge variation in the order of acquisition, depending on personality factors, experiences, modelling and the content of the AAC system. There is also a progression in complexity within each communication function: it is easier to simply say 'thank you' but saying 'I am so happy that you are in my life' is more sophisticated.

DOI: 10.4324/9781003296850-39

Earlier Communication Functions	Later Communication Functions
Request an action, person, object, help	Create social closeness
Protest or reject	Use manners
Greet or take leave	Sustain interaction
Name or label an object or action	End interaction
Give an answer	Express opinion
Comment	Express idea
Start or initiate interaction	Recall past experiences
Ask a concrete question (who, where, what)	Tell a story
Ask an abstract question (why, when, how)	Tell a pretend story
Express discomfort	Express emotion
Express appreciation or gratitude	Express hopes and dreams

PRAGMATIC ORGANISATION DYNAMIC DISPLAY (PODD)

This is an AAC approach which highlights the functions of language. Rather than vocabulary being organised by category, it is organised into functions like 'I'm telling you something', 'I'm asking a question' and 'I have an idea'. PODD can be used in communication books and is also available in AAC apps and vocabulary software. Modelling is a huge part of implementation. PODD training is highly recommended if this is an AAC solution you might use. Even if you are not directly providing PODD resources, the training is an excellent AAC training for SLTs developing a specialism in AAC.

THE IMPORTANCE OF MODELLING

We can't expect a child to use a communication function if it hasn't been modelled to them.

Often there is an objective set for a child to express their emotions, but how often is this modelled? If we want children to acquire this communication function, then they will need to regularly hear phrases like 'I'm so frustrated!' and 'I'm disappointed.'

TRACKING PROGRESS

Just like in spoken language development, it is useful to track a child's use of various communication functions. The SLT might ask a child's family or school to write down a sample of what they are saying to get an idea of which communication functions they are using and which might need to be developed.

ADULT PERSPECTIVES

We also need to consider communication functions with adult AAC users. If they have acquired speech difficulties because of stroke or head injury, then they once had the ability to express a range of communication functions. Just like with the child population, we don't want to focus entirely on getting wants and needs met. We also need to think about the communication functions that allow them to connect with others: creating social closeness, sustaining interaction, recalling past experiences, and so on. This goes beyond the here-and-now. We might build in phrases that consider the past or future, or that incorporate ideas, thoughts, wishes and regrets. For example 'Imagine if . . .' or 'I've been thinking about. . .'. We can work collaboratively with the AAC user to establish if these sorts of phrases would be appreciated.

CONVERSATION CLUB

WHY MIGHT WE NEED IT?

Conversations happen relatively easily for people who use natural speech. They can easily initiate a conversation around any topic. Once they have engaged another person, they can easily interject, add a brief word or two to keep the conversation going, repair misunderstandings, and so on.

Conversations are co-created. We don't know what we are going to say before a conversation starts. What we say is contingent upon what our conversation partner says. We go off on tangents. We add details and embelllish stories. We talk about our thoughts and feelings in response to what the other person says. We reminisce about the past and we fantasise about the future. At its best, conversation is a dynamic and highly creative process.

USING MULTI-MODAL COMMUNICATION

Conversations using AAC are more challenging. This is partly because of the speed of AAC communication. When we speak we generally create over 125 words per minute. AAC users tend to create one to eight words per minute.

However, the AAC user does not need to create full sentences to have fulfilling conversations. It is possible to have a creative, sparky conversation with an AAC user who supplies one or two-word phrases. An attuned conversation partner can co-create meaning from these. Sometimes a turn is non-verbal. So long as the conversation partner is monitoring the AAC user's multi-modal communication (including their

DOI: 10.4324/9781003296850-40

yes/no response, vocalisations, facial expressions, body language, gestures and signs), they can build rich conversations full of emotional nuance.

Take this extract from a conversation. Liz has noticed that Hannah has a theatre programme on the table in front of her.

Liz: 'Ooh – you have a Hamilton programme . . .'
Hannah: nods and her eyes light up.
Liz: 'Did you go to see it?'
Hannah: nodds vigorously, and holds hands to her heart.
Liz: looks to the communication book, and says 'Can you tell me about it?'
Hannah: pauses to think. They finger-spell 'B'.
Liz: 'Someone beginning with B – Bill? Your son? Or nephew?'
Hannah: nods and signs 'tall', looking up and looking surprised.
Liz: 'He's all grown up?'
Hannah: nods and gestures driving.
Liz: 'He drove you in his car?'
Hannah: nods and gestures holding onto the seat.
Liz: 'He drove fast?'

The conversation continued, with Hannah using a mixture of gesture, nodding, and using her communication book to add one or two more details each turn. The non-verbal communication, including facial expression and body language is highly descriptive. It effectively adds the tone of voice, adding nuance of meaning to enhance the generic nature of a symbol or word. I would argue that this emotional attunement, picking up on the feelings the person has about what they are telling you, is the most important part of a conversation. This is true connection between two people.

COMMUNICATION PARTNER TRAINING

Any conversation club will require a basic level of communication partner training, so that the conversation partners are attuned to all the ways an AAC user may add meaning to their message. See Chapter 12 for more information on conversation partner training.

CONVERSATION STOPPERS

Before considering how we start conversations, we should consider what stops a conversation. Asking too many closed questions, especially ones where we already know the answer, kills a conversation. Open questions offer more freedom, but they can also be overwhelming or pressurised. The classic question that parents ask their children at the end of the day is 'What did you do today?', and most children, regardless of communication ability, reply with a very brief answer. Adults struggle with this too. When we ask 'How are you?' we tend to give a stock phrase, like 'Very well thank you.'

INVITATIONAL LANGUAGE

Invitational language places a temptation to communicate. These are phrases that communicate that there is all the time in the world, and that a response is optional. There is no pressure, and there is definitely not a 'right' answer.

A sentence starter can be a non-threatening way to invite just a word or two. The communication partner starts the sentence, and then leaves space for the AAC user to complete it. 'You're working on . . .' 'You're thinking about . . .' 'You're worrying about. . .'. This requires the communication partner to be attuned to the AAC user's non-verbal communication, in order to know how to start the sentence. They also need to monitor the response, and to identify if they went down the wrong track.

A similar approach is to comment, rather than ask a question. For example, 'I see that . . .' (you have a new haircut, look worried, and so on)'. Or 'Your partner told me that . . . (you have struggled with the book this week, you are excited about tomorrow, and so on)'.

You might comment on the AAC user's non-verbal communication. For example, 'You look like you have something to say', 'You look worried,' or 'You're looking at the door.' This kind of phrase, said in a gentle way, lets them know that you see them. This is often enough to start a conversation.

My favourite invitational phrases start with wondering. For example 'I'm wondering how last week went' or 'I'm wondering if you have any thoughts on this'. This technique lends itself to having something to look at. For instance a photograph or a picture book. For example 'I wonder what happened here', 'I wonder what she is thinking' or 'I wonder how she is feeling.'

Notice that there is no question mark! A response is optional. Once you have said an invitational phrase, wait. Give the AAC user plenty of time to process what you have said, to decide if they want to respond, and formulate a response.

A final suggestion is a question, but there is an option to decline. It is 'Can you tell me about . . .?' You can also use 'Can you tell me *more about that*?' to invite further details. Again it is important that the communication partner monitors the non-verbal communication and spots any sign that they are not comfortable with this approach. If a mistake is made, then the communication partner apologises. For example 'I can see you don't want to talk about that right now', or 'It looks like you want to talk about something else.'

PLAYSCRIPTS AND ROLE PLAY

We may want the AAC user to practice using specific vocabulary, for instance core words and core phrases. We may want them to practice specific grammatical structures, like questions or negatives. We may want to target specific communciation functions, like asking directions, giving information to a health professional, or reporting a concern.

Playscripts and role play lend themselves to this. We may ask a group of AAC users which situations they struggle with, and then jointly write a playscript for how to manage it. The SLT might write up the script, using text or symbols, as appropriate. They may support the acting out of the script, providing appropriate prompts. These prompts may then be phased out, and the playscript may turn into a more spontaneous role play. The opportunity to improvise makes this more fun and promotes group bonding.

CONVERSATION STARTERS

Conversation using AAC can be enhanced by using resources to start the conversation.

Telling stories is perhaps the most important part of conversation: we love telling stories about what has happened to us, and also about what we would like to happen. Part of being a creative human being is to imagine 'what if'. Visual supports can promote this kind of creative conversation.

There are some excellent resources on the educational website 'Twinkl'. There are a whole range of illustrated conversational starters like:

- Would you rather explore under water or in outer space? Why?
- Would you rather take the bus or ride a bike? Why?
- Do you prefer summer or winter? Why?
- Would you rather paint or dance? Why?
- Do you prefer the city or the countryside? Why?
- Would you rather be invisible or be able to fly? Why?

For adults, you might ask more philosphical questions like:

- If you could go anywhere, where would it be?
- If you could talk to anyone for an hour, who would it be?
- If you could change one thing about the world, what would it be?
- Would you rather be young and inexperienced or old and wise? Why?
- What message would you tell your younger self?
- What would you like people in the future to know about you?

As some of these questions are very personal, it is advisable that people can choose to 'pass' on a question. You might ask for feedback about the types of conversation starters you are using. If you are running a conversation club, you could 'co-create' it with the AAC users, so that they suggest topics and help to design the activities.

LITERACY, LEARNING AND AAC

SYMBOLS OR TEXT?

THE BENEFITS OF SYMBOLS

Symbols are a visual way to represent language if an AAC user does not have basic literacy. Using an established symbol set is recommended. They have been carefully designed to be as representative of the word as possible, including key features, but not being overly specific so that they don't represent all forms of that word.

Symbol sets like WLS, PCS and Symbolstix have design themes that can help an AAC user build grammatical knowledge about pronouns, verbs, adjectives, prepositions and so on. For more about the different symbol sets, see Chapter 16.

THE LIMITATIONS OF SYMBOLS

In AAC resources, we always display the written word beneath or above the symbol. This helps the communication partner, as symbols often cannot be guessed easily from the symbol alone. People with good literacy often find reading quicker than trying to work out what a symbol means.

Symbols take up space on the page, and therefore a communication book using symbols will be bulky. They are also costly to print out, if they are printed in colour.

The vocabulary of a symbol-based AAC solution will be limited. A communication book or an AAC app may have a couple of thousand symbols, but the vocabulary of a speaking person is between 20,000 and 40,000 words.

Speaking people can use new words easily. They can even create their own new word if they can't think of one which works.

DOI: 10.4324/9781003296850-42

AAC users who use symbols can be creative: they can use a symbol in a different way, for example, using a noun as a verb or adjective, like 'you look rainbow' or 'stripe it'. If they don't have the exact word on their AAC solution they may be able to describe it. For example 'plug car' (electric car) or 'fat hairy plant' (cactus). But another option would be to spell it.

Some symbols, particularly the grammatical words, like 'the', 'and', 'but' and 'it' are so abstract that they may as well be represented by the text only. This is the recommendation for most AAC users who are learning literacy: if they have to learn an abstract shape, they may as well learn the whole word for the high-frequency core words.

Symbols can limit the progression of literacy, if in literacy activities the letters and words are always accompanied by symbols. It is a visual distraction, and the learner may look at the symbol more than they focus on the shape of the letter or the sight word.

THE BENEFITS OF LITERACY

We live in a literate world. Whilst it is true that signs, leaflets and posters, particularly if they have picture or symbol support, can give us basic information, we miss a lot of information too. Symbols do not have the specificity of written language. Try reading back a symbolised sentence: there may be multiple possible meanings, particularly around verb tenses, and whether it is a statement or a question.

Literacy opens up a whole world of language and learning. It gives us full access to the world around us. We can access books, magazines, newspapers, subtitles, social media, the internet, emails, text messages . . .

Until we have good functional literacy, we learn new words by hearing them. But once we are able to read, we acquire new vocabulary mainly by reading. We can direct our own learning, simply by choosing what to read.

Anyone can learn to read, even if they are much older than school age. Even if they have learning disabilities. Even if they have no spoken language. We may have to adapt the approach to teaching literacy, so that we focus on visual spelling patterns rather than phonics: you can read more about this in the next two chapters.

Of course, sometimes a stroke or head injury will mean that a person has lost their literacy. But they may have retained some literacy. Some literacy is better than none.

A COMBINATION OF SYMBOLS AND TEXT

If an AAC user has emerging literacy, or if the AAC user has lost literacy skills but retained some reading or spelling ability, then a combination of symbols or text may work well.

High-frequency core words like pronouns, articles and prepositions might be represented by text alone.

An alphabet chart or page will give access to spelling. Even spelling the first one or two letters can really help a communication partner to guess a word, or prediction software can then offer suggestions for the rest of the word. See Chapter 21 for more information about alphabet charts.

RECOMMENDED RESOURCES

The ACE Centre have a range of free downloadable alphabet charts which can be used in communication books or on the reverse of a communication board.

Karen Erickson has done more to further the cause of literacy for AAC users than any other professional. Her book *Comprehensive Literacy for All*[1] sets out her strategies for making literacy teaching accessible for non-verbal students.

For an introduction to teaching literacy to AAC users, the Kent and Medway Communication and Assistive Technology (KM CAT) service have developed training and eLearning to put Karen Erickson's ideas into a practical UK-based model for teaching. See their website for details.

CASE STUDY: KADEN'S PROGRESSION FROM SYMBOLS TO TEXT

Kaden started off with a symbolised communication book and vocabulary package on an iPad. He got to know these two AAC solutions very well by the time he started school.

Kaden was given an alphabet chart and an alphabet page on his vocabulary package from the time he started school. During all lessons (not just literacy) teaching staff would show Kaden how to spell sight words and would help him to learn the sounds and letters of the alphabet. Kaden would identify the first and last letters in CVC (consonant-vowel-consonant) words, and then he progressed to CVCC, and CCVC words, and so on.

In Kaden's symbolised communication book and his vocabulary package on his VOCA, it was decided to remove the symbols for the core words. These were also the sight words that he was learning in his literacy lessons. Kaden could do matching activities so that when flashcards were used, he matched them to the relevant core word on his VOCA.

Kaden's parents read picture books to him each evening. They also pointed out print in the environment: when they were driving in the car, when they were at the supermarket, on the television and computer, and so on.

Kaden had prediction software on his AAC vocabulary package which meant he could start to spell a word and then could choose the target words from one of the 4 prediction cells on the screen. It was decided that symbolised prediction did not allow him to look at the letters and word shapes, and so the symbols were removed from the prediction cells.

By Year 5, Kaden preferred to use his alphabet chart or alphabet page on his vocabulary package, rather than his symbolised pages. He had also programmed some stored text-based messages on his VOCA and used these in everyday conversation. Over the next two years he transitioned into using text only.

NOTE

1 Erickson, K. and Koppenhaver, D. *Comprehensive Literacy for All: Teaching Students with Significant Disabilities to Read and Write*, Brookes Publishing, 2020.

ASSESSING LITERACY

HOW CAN WE ASSESS A NON-SPEAKING CHILD'S LITERACY?

It is generally perceived to be much harder to assess and teach literacy if a child has no speech. These children can't 'sound out' phonemes or read aloud sight words. This is not a barrier to learning literacy: it just means that assessment will depend more on offering choices, rather like a multiple-choice test, and the child will have to choose the correct option. Partner-assisted scanning is an excellent technique for assessing literacy (and all learning).

WHO SHOULD ASSESS AND TEACH LITERACY?

It is recommended that the SLT liaises closely with the teacher, to make sure that there is a shared understanding that it is still possible to assess and teach literacy. The SLT may signpost the teacher to training (see the Recommended Resources section of this chapter)

A FRAMEWORK FOR ASSESSING LITERACY LEVELS

In *Comprehensive Literacy for All*, Erickson and Koppenhaver set out a framework for assessing and teaching literacy.[1]

They ask us to answer four questions about a child's literacy: These are shown on the following page.

Once we know whether they need 'emergent' or 'conventional' literacy teaching, we focus on the interventions listed above. These will be explored in more detail in the following chapter.

Just like AAC intervention, we need everyone to be on board with literacy teaching. We need the teaching staff, but

DOI: 10.4324/9781003296850-43

1. Can the student identify most of the letters of the alphabet, most of the time?
2. Is the student engaged and interactive during shared reading?
3. Does the student have a means of communication and interaction?
4. Does the student understand that print has meaning?

'NO' to one or more questions	'YES' to all questions
Step 1 emergent literacy teaching	**Step 2** conventional literacy teaching
1 Shared reading 2 Shared writing 3 Alphabet and phonological awareness 4 Independent writing with access to the full alphabet 5 Self-directed reading	1 Reading comprehension 2 Word study 3 Writing 4 Self-directed reading

we also need parents and carers to be reinforcing literacy at home. Children need daily literacy teaching; formal and informal. We need a coordinated approach so that literacy skills are taught and assessed in a systematic way, with revision built in. Fortunately, we now have the resources to guide this.

RECOMMENDED RESOURCES

As previously recommended, the ACE Centre have a range of free downloadable alphabets charts which can be used in communication books or on the reverse of a communication board.

Erickson and Koppenhaver's book *Comprehensive Literacy for All*[2] sets out the strategies for making literacy teaching accessible for non-verbal students.

For an introduction to teaching literacy to AAC users, the Kent and Medway Communication and Assistive Technology (KM CAT) service have developed training and eLearning to put Karen Erickson's ideas into a practical UK-based model for teaching. See their website for details.

CASE STUDY: JEMIMA'S ALPHABET

Jemima was assessed informally using the framework above. It was found that she didn't yet know most of her letters.

The SLT agreed with Jemima's teacher and parents that they would revise groups of 6 letters per day in a cyclical and systematic way so that every letter was revised every week for the next eight weeks. The adults were free to be creative in the way they revised letters. They could add the six letters to a sand tray, put them in a feely bag, hide them in the bath, write them on balloons, make an alphabet book, and so on.

By the end of eight weeks, Jemima knew most of the letters most of the time. She could accurately point to a named letter from a choice of six letters. This was also how her paper-based alphabet chart was arranged, with letters grouped so that they could be more easily located. Jemima had access to this alphabet chart throughout the day, not just in her literacy lessons.

Since Jemima already had a means of communication, an interest in shared reading and an understanding that print carries meaning, she was now ready for daily conventional literacy teaching.

NOTES

1 Adapted from p. 201 of Erickson, K. and Koppenhaver, D. *Comprehensive Literacy for All: Teaching Students with Significant Disabilities to Read and Write*, Brookes Publishing, 2020.
2 Erickson, K. and Koppenhaver, D. *Comprehensive Literacy for All: Teaching Students with Significant Disabilities to Read and Write*, Brookes Publishing, 2020.

TEACHING LITERACY

WHO SHOULD TEACH LITERACY?

Whilst the teacher will have ultimate responsibility, everyone who interacts with a child has a role to play in their literacy development. Literacy teaching should not be restricted to literacy lessons. It should be incorporated into every subject so that the child gets repeated opportunities to apply skills throughout the school day.

Literacy teaching comes into virtually all daily activities too. Whether it is reading environmental print and pointing out the letters and sounds in packaging, logos, road signs and clothing. Or writing lists and notes for everyday activities. The more a child is exposed to talking about text, the quicker they will attain functional literacy.

EMERGENT LITERACY TEACHING

In the previous chapter, we looked at a framework for assessing literacy, developed by Erickson and Koppenhaver. What follows here are the activities to build these skills, in order to move a child from emergent literacy to conventional literacy. Erickson and Kopenhaver's book *Comprehensive Literacy for All*[1] is highly recommended for further detail.

1. SHARED READING

The emphasis in shared reading is on enjoying books together. First books can be entirely picture-based. This encourages genuine interaction between and adult and child, as they make meaning together. The child will get experience of initiating and responding and creating a possible story together. The adult can make links between the book and real life, for example, 'Do you remember when we went to the seaside?' The adult can use lots of invitational language, like 'I wonder what he is doing?' or simply 'uh-oh!'

Picture books with text can also be introduced. The adult might point out specific letters or words that are meaningful for the child. For example, the first letter of their name, or a repeated word. They might then encourage the child to find this letter or word and join in with reading the text. Books with rhyming patterns or repeated refrains are great for this. Favourites of mine include *Dear Zoo, Mr Magnolia, Hairy Mclary* and *We're Going on a Bear Hunt.*

2.   SHARED WRITING

Emergent writing is creative and fun. Scribbling and drawing gradually shapes itself into writing. A range of writing tools are provided: pens, pencils, crayons, chalks, markers, finger paint, sand, alphabet sets, and so on.

If a child cannot physically access these resources, then we can provide other tools to play around with letters and text. For example, a keyboard, onscreen keyboard accessed via a mouse, or a paper-based alphabet chart.

At first, the letter selections will be random, just as a child with a pencil will scribble. Gradually though, letters might be grouped together into word shapes. It is important that the adult assumes that these are meaningful and asks the child what they have written. The child can be creative in their interpretation. The important thing is that we are assuming competence: that this child has the intention to be literate, and can be proud of their attempts.

These writing attempts can even be made into books with pictures. This shows the child that their writing is valued.

This stage might include 'predictable chart writing', whereby the adult writes a repeated sentence with a gap in it. For example 'I like playing with . . .'. A group of children will each be encouraged to supply a word to fill the gap. Children can use their AAC or an alphabet chart to supply a word. Predictable chart writing teaches sentence structure and makes it easy for a child to feel the pleasure of creative writing.

3.   ALPHABET AND PHONOLOGICAL AWARENESS

In this stage, lower- and upper-case letters need to be presented in different sizes and fonts. Adults will need to keep naming them and saying their sound. Various alphabet tools and materials should be used to make this fun. For example, printing with letters, making cookies with letters, making snake letters from playdough, finding letters buried in sand, using alphabet books and songs, and having a collection of items which start with a specific letter or sound. Because the child who uses AAC is unlikely to be able to say the letter name and sound, the adults can encourage them to 'say it in your head'.

The child may be encouraged to search for a specific letter in text. They might also write or type a specific letter. They can use their AAC to do this: if they use an E-Tran frame, they can eye-point to the named letter. If they use partner-assisted auditory scanning, they can indicate 'yes' when the target letter is read out. If they use switch-scanning, they can hit their switch when the scanner gets to the target letter.

It is suggested that 'letter of the week' is ditched, because this means letter and sound learning is too slow (it would take 26 weeks to go through the alphabet). Erickson and Koppenhaver recommend that there is a 'letter of the day' instead, so that the letters are regularly revised and repeated.

Creating an alphabet book, either paper-based or screen-based, is a more active process than just reading alphabet books. These can be regularly revised and repeated. This might be something that the family enjoy doing too.

The phonological awareness skills of syllable-segmentation, rhyme awareness and alliteration are really important at this stage. Syllables can be clapped, stamped, drummed or rocked.

4.   INDEPENDENT WRITING WITH ACCESS TO THE FULL ALPHABET

AAC users should have access to a full alphabet, so that they can practice their literacy throughout the day in all activities and lessons. They should have access to a paper-based alphabet chart. They might access this using direct selection with their finger, fist or eye-pointing, or it may involve partner-assisted scanning.

They can also use technology to write. The child may be able to access a standard keyboard, but a small child-sized keyboard is recommended. A key-guard may be necessary to avoid accidental selections. If the child cannot access a keyboard, then an onscreen keyboard can be used. This might be accessed using an alternative mouse, like a joystick or rollerball, or with switch-scanning or eye-gaze technology. An OT will need to advise on the best access method (see Chapter 8).

There should be frequent opportunities to use writing throughout the day. No matter what lesson is being taught, a child can be encouraged to label pictures, write captions and write notes or lists.

5.   SELF-DIRECTED READING

Children are more likely to engage with books if they have completely free choice of reading material. This may be picture books, story books, factual books, magazines, comics, online books, or even catalogues, websites and videos with captions.

The child may choose a text which is either way below or way above their current reading level. This is ok: the adult can still support their reading attempts of the text. Conversation around what they did or didn't enjoy is also part of the reading experience. Children might share what they have been reading during group time with peers.

The child can be encouraged to follow the text with an adult. If it is an online book, the text being spoken might be highlighted. This encourages independent reading and reading for pleasure.

CONVENTIONAL LITERACY TEACHING

Referring back to the 'Framework for Assessing Literacy' in the previous chapter, once you can answer 'yes' to the four questions, the child can move on to conventional literacy teaching. In Erickson and Koppenhaver's method, these are the typical components of conventional literacy teaching:

1. READING COMPREHENSION

Adults might set a purpose to reading a given piece of text. The child will be asked to find out a piece of information which can only be gleaned from reading the text, like 'What different fruits did Handa carry in her basket?' The child might then apply this knowledge to an activity or piece of work. For example, they might write a shopping list or write a recipe to make a fruit salad.

2. WORD STUDY

AAC users who have no natural speech are going to find phonics very challenging because they can't 'sound out'.

We can use word families to show rhyming and spelling patterns, e.g. m-ake, c-ake, t-ake, b-ake, r-ake. This use of 'rime and onset' is more visual than synthetic phonics: the child can see the pattern. The first letter, or onset, might be detachable from the rest of the word, or rime. For example, there may be two puzzle pieces or Duplo blocks. We can show that the onset can be removed and replaced with a different onset.

We can build on the work around word families and 'rime-and-onset'. Either component might be manipulated, removing and replacing it with different letters to make a new word.

We might also compare and contrast two different word families, noticing the rime spelling pattern. The emphasis is on children actively engaging with the spelling pattern: what do they notice? What is the same or different about two different words?

The most common spelling patterns in English are shown below. Systematic teaching of each of these spelling patterns will allow a child to read at least 500 words.

ack	ail	ap	ash	aw	ale	ake
ate	ay	ank	an	ain	ame	all
eat	ell	ice	ide	it	ick	ip
ight	ill	in	ing	op	ot	oke
ore	ock	uck	ug	ump	est	ink
at	unk					

Word families can be played with as 3D objects. The onset and rime might be shown on giant dice or a spinner. An alphabet chart or onscreen keyboard can be used for these activities: a child who uses AAC might use their alphabet chart to choose the onset, and later the rime, or to spell the whole word.

Words might be sorted into their word families, for example –ay and –unk words. Later, the child might be asked to generate words for a word family when they are given the rime. An alphabet chart or onscreen keyboard can be used for this.

Sight words are high-frequency words which often have irregular spellings. It is helpful to have a systematic order for learning these, with regular revision built in. A 'word wall' might be built to reflect the sight words that have been learnt. The spelling patterns of sight words might be used to spell other words, for example 'look' relates to 'book'; the letters and sound in 'the' are the same as in 'this', 'that', 'though' and so on.

If these activities can be blended with other lessons and daily activities, all the better. Literacy comes into every lesson, and will be acquired faster if the skills are reinforced across the curriculum.

3.   WRITING

Adults can help the creative process by providing a topic for writing. There may be a photo book of interesting images meant to provide inspiration for writing. Starter questions like 'If you could go anywhere, where would it be?' or 'If you were an animal, what would you be?' can be helpful.

It is helpful to establish a culture of 'writing without worrying'. First drafts should be free from rules about spelling, grammar and punctuation.

It is helpful for the adult to ask the child to read their text back to them. The adult can then make a positive comment about the content (rather than the form), like 'I'm scared of thunder too. I wonder if anyone else is?' This demonstrates to the child that their writing is meaningful and promotes connection with others.

4.   SELF-DIRECTED READING

This will continue to build on the interests of the child. They should be exposed to as wide a choice of texts as possible.

Reading time can be made fun and indulgent. It could accompany a snack. There could be a reading picnic area, or a reading tent. The reading space should be as inviting as possible. A timer might be used for reluctant readers. One minute of looking at a book is a realistic first step.

If adults take an interest in the child's reading choices, this is likely to increase their motivation to read. Celebrating their reading is likely to be more motivating than an extrinsic reward. The child might have regular scheduled conversations with the teacher about their reading choices.

RECOMMENDED RESOURCES

The ACE Centre have a range of free downloadable alphabets charts with a range of layouts and access options.

Erickson and Koppenhaver's book *Comprehensive Literacy for All* sets out this systematic method for teaching literacy to non-verbal students.

For an introduction to teaching literacy to AAC users, the Kent and Medway Communication and Assistive Technology

CASE STUDY: RITIK'S WRITING

Ritik is eight years old. He has a partner-assisted auditory scanning communication book.

Ritik had been assessed as needing emergent literacy teaching. He previously had no way of mark-making or 'writing' because of his physical disabilities.

The OT worked with Ritik and set up a laptop with a joystick and an onscreen keyboard. Ritik was then allowed to play with the onscreen keyboard. Adults encouraged him to make captions for photos, write notes to his friends, and make lists of things for the adults to remember. Adults responded to all of Ritik's typing positively and asked him about his writing. Ritik could use his communication book to tell adults the words he had typed.

Over the next few weeks, adults noticed that when Ritik was 'typing', he was grouping letters into 'words', with spaces between. He showed a preference for the letter 'R'. His teaching assistant helped him to make a whole book with 'R' words, with photos and pictures from the internet. Ritik then captioned these. Soon he was asking the adult how the word was spelt and trying to find the right letter with his onscreen keyboard.

Ritik's class were systematically taught the letters and sounds of the alphabet over the next academic year. Ritik was able to choose the onset in 'onset and rime' word family games.

Ritik went on to make many more mini books, leaflets, notes and lists. He was also able to access 'Clicker' software in order to show his learning in lessons. This also allowed Ritik to use the text-to-speech function, so that he could listen back to his work and make corrections.

(KM CAT) service have developed training and eLearning to put Erickson and Koppenhaver's ideas into a practical UK-based model for teaching. See their website for details.

NOTE

1 Erickson, K. and Koppenhaver, D. *Comprehensive Literacy for All: Teaching Students with Significant Disabilities to Read and Write*, Brookes Publishing, 2020.

ACCESS TO THE CURRICULUM

The child or young person will have a teaching team working with them, which may include a specialist teacher for physical, learning or sensory disabilities. Whilst it is the responsibility of the school to make education accessible, the SLT may contribute to giving advice about how to do this. The SLT will give advice about how to make spoken language more accessible, and how to model and support the use of AAC in the classroom.

Common SLCN (Speech, Language and Communication Needs) strategies apply here, such as making learning interactive, multi-sensory and meaningful, slowing down, chunking information, providing visual support, and building in regular review and revision of material.

There are also some more specific AAC strategies and resources detailed below.

TOPIC OR SUBJECT-SPECIFIC VOCABULARY

Topic or subject-specific vocabulary does not necessarily need adding to the student's AAC system. If it is only needed for a few weeks, a paper-based topic vocabulary sheet may be used to supplement the student's AAC system. This may or may not need to be symbolised, depending on the needs of the student.

When a student is in secondary education, they may have dedicated pages for each subject. This should include links to existing relevant vocabulary. For example, a 'Biology' page might have words like 'photosynthesis' and also have links to pages like 'animals', 'plants' and 'the body'.

DOI: 10.4324/9781003296850-45

If the student has sufficient literacy, they may spell out these subject-specific words. Using prediction software will be helpful to reduce fatigue. They may also store whole phrases, for example for English literature quotations.

TAKING PART IN DISCUSSIONS

It will be helpful if the teaching staff are familiar with a student's AAC solution. The SLT may offer some level of training (see 'Communcation partner training' in Chapter 12).

If the student can indicate 'yes' and 'no' then they can answer immediate verbal questions in class. The teacher may also give the student limited options in order to answer a quick question. For example: 'What do we call it when a liquid becomes a gas? Is it evaporation [pause] or condensation [pause]?'

The teacher will also ask open questions. The student might receive these in advance, or they may be given extra time to answer the question in class. All students might be asked to formulate a response in this way, maybe writing their answer whilst the AAC user is creating their response using their AAC.

ASSESSMENT OF LEARNING

Teachers carry out frequent assessments of students' learning, and sometimes express concern that they cannot assess an AAC user's learning. AAC users can be assessed if questions are structured in a multiple-choice format. The options may be read out, using partner-assisted auditory scanning. They may be offered as a visual choice, in a paper-based or screen-based format. They may be offered on an E-Tran frame.

SOFTWARE TO SUPPORT WRITTEN RECORDING

AAC solutions are primarily for spoken language. However, there is also a need for written work to show learning. This is known as 'written recording'.

Many AAC users will not be able to record their learning using a pen and pencil, because of their physical difficulties.

These students are often allocated a scribe: a person who writes down their ideas for them. This is not ideal. It requires extra processing to be able to tell another person your ideas as you are formulating them. It is also not helpful in terms of independence.

A better solution is to use software that enables the student to independently record their work. 'Clicker' is a programme that allows students to do this. Younger students might match words or sentences to pictures. They might fill in a missing gap in a sentence, or they may order all the words in a sentence. There is a 'screen-reader' function where they can click on a word and it will be spoken aloud. Students can progress to typing words, with a 'talking predictor' as an option. 'Word banks' can be used for topic vocabulary whereby the student selects a word from a given word bank. Word banks can be arranged by sub-topic or alphabetically, if the student's literacy permits.

'Docs Plus' is an equivalent programme for literate students, geared towards secondary education. It has many of the same features as 'Clicker' but does not rely on using pictures alongside text. It allows the student to create mind maps and use writing frames for more in-depth pieces of writing. Students can work with other documents, such as worksheets or exam papers, within the programme. 'Docs Plus' has an 'exam mode' which enables students to take formal exams like GCSEs and A Levels whilst using the programme.

ESTABLISHING A 'NORMAL WAY OF WORKING' FOR EXAM ACCESS

It is important that the student establishes these 'normal ways or working' early in their secondary education. This is so that the school can apply to the exam board to describe what the student uses to show their learning. This includes the use of AAC, topic vocabulary sheets or curriculum software such as 'Docs Plus'. The student will then be allowed to use their AAC and any curriculum software to access exams.

RECOMMENDED RESOURCES

'Clicker' and 'Docs Plus' software can be explored on Crick's website. There are short videos which demonstrate the programmes. Free trials are usually available. Schools may purchase site licences so that the whole school, including parents at home, can use the software.

CASE STUDY: DAN'S INDEPENDENT LEARNING

Dan uses a communication book and a tablet VOCA with a vocabulary package. His teachers provide a vocabulary list at the start of a topic, and his TA creates a symbolised version. Dan can then create sentences using his usual AAC and the symbolised topic chart. Dan's TA often scribes for him, but this doesn't give him the independence he needs.

Dan began to use Clicker, accessing this on a laptop, using a joystick. He found word-to-picture matching easy, and so quickly moved on to selecting words in the right order to make a sentence. Soon Dan was creating his own sentences. He used his AAC and his symbolised topic chart for copying spellings. His TA recognised that he was ready to use 'word banks' and so these were created in place of his symbolised topic chart.

Within a year, Dan was able to use word banks and typing with prediction to create his own pieces of writing.

ADVOCACY
AND AAC

TALKING MATS

WHAT ARE THEY?

Talking Mats are a visual communication framework for talking to people with communication difficulties about issues which concern them. This may inform person-centred planning. It also supports safeguarding and work around Mental Capacity.

The issues which might be explored include health and wellbeing, social care, keeping safe and thinking ahead. A Talking Mats session is scripted and structured to facilitate people with learning disabilities or cognitive impairment to process complex issues and express their genuine thoughts and feelings in a safe way.

Talking Mats provide the materials, which may be purchased as an app or as a physical mat with sets of pictures. The pictures are deliberately not symbols: they contain rich semantic details, including facial expressions, body language and environmental details which may trigger associations in their real life.

To carry out a Talking Mat, the facilitator must be trained in the Talking Mats approach.

A Talking Mat consists of three types of picture. The first shows the topic, at the top of the mat, for example 'Home'. Then there is a 'top scale' of three options, for example 'going well' on the left, 'not going well' on the right, and in the middle, 'sometimes going well'. The facilitator then shows pictures, one at a time, which the person can place under 'going well', 'not going well' or 'sometimes going well'. For the topic of 'Home' these might include 'getting in and out', 'maintenance and repairs', 'safety inside', 'safety outside', 'neighbours' and so on.

If the person cannot physically place the picture, then the facilitator will offer each of the three options in turn and place the picture for them. The facilitator will invite the person to say more. At the end, the facilitator asks the person to review where the pictures are. They can be changed if the person is not happy. A photo is then taken of the mat.

It is likely that a Talking Mat will need to be followed up with agreed actions. For example a problem may have been identified with 'maintenance and repairs' which needs to be raised with the key worker.

HOW DO THEY HELP?

Talking Mats offer the visual structure that people with communication difficulties need in order to explore complex issues. They break complex issues down into manageable, concrete chunks. They reduce processing and memory demands. Skilled facilitation can reduce anxiety, and may free the person from a tendency to 'people please'.

There is a record of this discussion and agreed actions. This ensures accountability to a service-user. They are genuinely involved in decision-making and care-planning.

WHO DO THEY HELP?

- Adults and children with learning disabilities and cognitive impairment who can understand beyond the 'here and now'.

RECOMMENDED RESOURCES

See the website for a wealth of information about Talking Mats. Videos are included, so that you can see a Talking Mat in action.

CASE STUDY: HELEN'S TALKING MAT FOR PLANNING TREATMENT

Helen has Multiple Sclerosis. At the moment she is coping well, but she wants to make plans for when her health deteriorates.

An SLT came to meet Helen and they completed a Talking Mat around her 'Care and Treatment Wishes'. This allowed Helen to think about how much medical intervention she wanted, how she wanted to be fed and hydrated, and where she wanted to be cared for at the end of her life.

Through completing the Talking Mat, Helen identified that she was worried about her daughter, particularly if nutrition was withdrawn. The SLT agreed actions with Helen, which included offering a session with Helen's daughter to discuss these issues. She could also be referred to counselling to support her.

Helen reported that she felt relieved at the end of the Talking Mats sessions. She had been aware that this issue had been causing her stress, but had not been able to get her thoughts straight. Breaking the topics down into each small component was very helpful. Helen felt that she was given the time to think, and she liked that there were specific actions that were followed up after the Talking Mats session.

Helen kept the photo of her Talking Mat, and later used these when she talked to her daughter. A detailed report was written by the SLT and this informed an advance decision for Helen's end of life care.

42

MENTAL CAPACITY AND MAKING DECISIONS

WHAT IS MENTAL CAPACITY?

Mental capacity describes a person's ability to make a decision about their health or social care. They may need support to make a decision, and the information they are given may be modified to enable them to understand the information, weigh up the pros and cons, retain the information, and make an informed decision. Individuals have the right to make a decision that their family, carers or professionals do not agree with. In England and Wales, people over the age of 16 have the right to make decisions. Sometimes children under the age of 16 have capacity: it depends upon the decision.

Some individuals lack capacity for some decisions. They may be currently unable to make a decision because of illness, stress, lack of sleep or food, social pressure, medication or substance misuse. The timing is important: when we are assessing mental capacity, we are only assessing for this decision at this time. A person may lack capacity for some decisions, but they will be able to make other decisions. It depends on the complexity of the decision.

BUILDING DECISION-MAKING SKILLS

Decision-making is a skill that we start to develop from when we are very young. As toddlers we start to make our own decisions: which toy to pick up, where to crawl, what to eat, whether to comply with a request, and so on. This is the start of independence and a sense of agency and competence. Children are gradually trusted to make more complex decisions: what to

DOI: 10.4324/9781003296850-48

wear, who to play with, which toy they want for Christmas, who to invite to their birthday party.

There will be some decisions that young people need support with, for instance, managing spending money, what GCSEs to choose, a suitable bed-time, and so on. Adults can help to support decision-making by offering the options, discussing pros and cons and maybe providing some visual structure to help them retain the information. An important part of the process is making a few bad decisions. This helps us learn about the consequences of our decisions. If we spend all our money on an app, there is none left for make-up. If we choose History GCSE, we are signed up for two years.

Children with physical, sensory or learning disabilities may not get so many opportunities to make decisions in this way. They may become used to others making choices for them. We therefore need to make sure that decision-making is built into their AAC intervention, so that they get used to making increasingly complex decisions.

It has been estimated that we make around 35000 decisions per day. Some are very simple and we barely notice them. Some decisions are big, and we may make weeks or months to make them. Our personal preferences, emotions, knowledge and values will come into decision-making. Decision-making is not so much about choosing the 'right' option, but the option that is right for us at this time.

AAC AND DECISION-MAKING

To make a decision, we need to be able to:

1. Understand the information relevant to the decision.
2. Retain the information.
3. Think about the information, and weigh up the pros and cons.
4. Communicate the decision.

AAC can play a role in all four of these steps. A decision and the options may be supported with visual supports. These may be used to assess whether a person has remembered what the decision is about: they may point to a symbol or word that represents the decision, e.g. 'house' or 'medicine'. They may be given an 'easy read' or symbolised summary of the pros and cons, and asked to point to what is good or bad about an option, e.g. 'sleepiness', 'no pain'. They then also need to be given a means of communicating their choice. This may be a simple 'yes' or 'no' or it may need to be more nuanced. 'I'm not sure' should always be an option. There should also be an option to request 'something else'.

For AAC users who are cognitively able and have good receptive language, we do not need to go through a lengthy process of checking that they have understood: we should give them accessible information which explains pros and cons, and then seek their consent with them using their AAC. If we know the individual well enough, we should have a good idea about their capacity.

IF THE PERSON LACKS CAPACITY

If a person lacks capacity for an important decision regarding their health or social care, then a 'best interests' decision may be made. In England and Wales, the Mental Capacity Act (MCA) sets out how capacity should be assessed. The person's preferences, emotions and values need to be taken into consideration: what is right for one person is not necessarily right for another. The person's human rights are always of paramount importance, including the rights for freedom of thought, conscience and religion, the right not to be discriminated against, and the right to liberty.

RECOMMENDED RESOURCES

You can read about the Mental Capacity Act on the government website. There is an easy read version on the local government website. Dorset County Council have produced an animated video which can be found on video streaming platforms.

CASE STUDY: JUDE'S DECISION

Jude is 17 years old. They have always had difficulties with their eating and have had a modified texture diet. Their parents preferred oral feeding, particularly from a social perspective.

Jude has been steadily losing weight and is lacking in energy. The SLT felt that, given Jude's age, it was time to revisit the management plan.

Jude uses a symbolised communication book. They understand 3 information-carrying words if the sentence is supported with symbols. They understand basic concepts, including some concepts of time, and can talk beyond the 'here and now'.

The SLT prepared an information sheet, which set out the options for Jude, including continuing with a modified texture diet, or being PEG fed, or a combination of both. This showed the pros and cons of each option.

Jude could show that they understood the information. When the SLT asked what was good about each option, Jude could point to relevant symbols. For example, for the option of modified texture, that there was a risk of 'coughing' and getting 'ill'. For PEG feeding, Jude pointed to 'hospital' and that the stoma needed a 'dressing'.

The SLT told Jude that they could think about the options and that they would talk about them again in a week.

In the second session, Jude demonstrated that they had retained the information. When Jude was asked if they knew which option they preferred, Jude pointed to the 'PEG' option. The SLT used Jude's communication book to reiterate that this would mean 'no eating' and 'no drinking'. Jude nodded and again pointed to 'PEG'. Jude then said 'no eat ok'.

The team around Jude concluded that Jude had capacity to make this decision, and Jude went ahead with PEG feeding.

43

SAFEGUARDING AND AAC

WHAT ROLE DOES AAC HAVE IN SAFEGUARDING?

Individuals who have a communication impairment are more vulnerable to abuse, neglect, exploitation or a crime being committed against them. We can help reduce the risk by building communication skills that reduce their vulnerability.

VOCABULARY FOR SAFEGUARDING

Core vocabulary is important for reporting a concern. For example, 'I not like' or 'not want go'.

In addition, it is helpful if an AAC user can identify the names of people. Being able to spell the first letter in a name is useful.

They also need access to everyday verbs and parts of the body. We should be promoting the anatomically accurate names of body parts. By shying away from terms like 'vulva' we are promoting silence and confusion.

Safeguarding is not about making a person feel scared, but about making them feel empowered. We need to provide vocabulary around periods, sexual health, relationships and sexual pleasure. We are empowering the individual if they know how their body functions and what they can expect from a healthy relationship.

It takes practice to accurately describe bodily sensations such as being 'hot', 'cold', 'uncomfortable', 'hungry', 'thirsty' or 'tired'. Pain might be described as 'sharp', 'dull', or 'achy'. Visual supports might help to teach these concepts. Rating scales might be introduced for levels of pain or sensation. If an AAC user is used to doing this in their daily care, they can then report concerns if their care is not what it ought to be.

 DOI: 10.4324/9781003296850-49

COMMUNICATION FUNCTIONS FOR SAFEGUARDING

We need to build frequent opportunities for making choices, so that the AAC user is used to having agency. In choice-making, it is important to include the option of 'something else'. We can move on to the skill of being able to say 'no' or 'something's wrong'. This can be taught in a fun way. For example, the adult might ask silly questions, like 'Is this a giraffe?' (holding a picture of an elephant). We might talk about 'What's wrong?' pictures, starting with concrete examples, and building into social scenarios involving thoughts and feelings.

Children and adults with disabilities are at risk of being 'people pleasers' because they are dependent on others for care. It is important that they get the opportunity to safely reject an option. Practice can begin with rejecting an item, and progress to rejecting an idea or opinion. There may need to be discussion that it is ok to feel differently to a friend or carer. For example, some people like dogs and some don't, but that's ok. We can say no to an activity with a person we like without them being cross with us. Social stories can be helpful for this work.

STORY-TELLING

Story-telling is an important skill. We might start with simple retelling of what we did in an activity, and then we might use sequencing pictures to tell a story. Stories might be selected which focus on asking for help when something goes wrong. We can use stories to talk about emotions. Fairy tales or soap operas might be useful sources for story retelling and talking about emotions.

GIVING AN OPINION

We should encourage AAC users to give their opinion at every opportunity. This helps to redress the power imbalance that occurs between a caregiver and receiver. We need to make it safe for someone to tell us when they are not happy with their care. After each appointment, we should be asking their opinion, using visual supports. We might use a rating scale or we might ask the person to give us a word or phrase to describe the session. We are building the expectation that their opinion is valued and that complaints will be acted upon.

DECISION-MAKING SKILLS

A person who is used to having agency, who is used to being consulted and who is used to consent being sought, is far less vulnerable to abuse. Decision-making skills can develop from simple decisions about what to wear, what to eat or drink, and what music or video to play. Intermediate decision-making might involve spending money, planning an event, or choosing leisure options. More complex decisions are those that involve housing, work, health or social care options. Visual supports can help with weighing up options in more complex decisions. See Chapter 41 on Talking Mats too.

SEEKING CONSENT

It is important that all those working with a person seek consent to carry out personal care. It will be obvious to the individual if someone is behaving differently and not respecting these boundaries. Recognising that something is wrong is the first step to being able to report a concern.

RESPONDING TO NON-VERBAL COMMUNICATION

As we discussed in Chapters 10 and 12, we should be noting and commenting on non-verbal communication, so that the AAC user sees that we are attuned to this. The AAC user will learn that they can corroborate or clarify an AAC message with their non-verbal communication.

REPORTING CONCERNS

A communication book or vocabulary package may have a specific page for reporting concerns. This might include a general 'something's wrong' or 'something happened'. There might be links to other pages of vocabulary, such as verbs to describe interaction, body parts, people and places.

Just as with any disclosure, the person recording the concern should ask open questions as much as possible. It is important to establish the who, what, when and where of a situation, if the AAC user is able to understand these questions. Partner-assisted scanning might be used, whereby the AAC user selects from options, or indicates 'yes' or 'no' to questions. There will need to be some way of recording what the person has said, using verbatim transcription, or a photo. Actions should be agreed with the AAC user.

RECOMMENDED RESOURCES

Social Stories, developed by Carol Gray, are an excellent way of teaching children and vulnerable adults about strategies to solve problems. They can also be used to reinforce expectations of how other people should behave and what to do if there is a problem. See Carol Gray's website for more information about social stories.

Talking Mats, discussed in Chapter 41, can be used as a tool to support advocacy and safeguarding.

Grid 3's vocabulary package, Voco Chat, has some useful pages which support safeguarding. There are pages devoted to 'something's wrong', 'Can I tell you something?' and 'Can I ask you something?' There are also pages relating to bodily sensations, emotions and strategies for self-care, and a rating scale so that the AAC user can give feedback to others about their wellbeing or the standard of care.

CASE STUDY: DOMINIC'S CONCERNS

Dominic lives in a shared house for adults with disabilities. A staff member noticed that Dominic was not his usual self. She asked him if something was wrong. Dominic indicated 'yes'. The staff member then encouraged Dominic to use his communication book to tell her more.

Dominic used his core words page to say 'no' and then turned to the 'house' page to say 'door'. The staff member said 'no door', and Dominic nodded. He looked towards the bathroom. The staff member was initially confused and thought about this. She then said 'You're upset about the bathroom door?' Dominic nodded. 'Did somebody leave the bathroom door open?' Dominic nodded and put his hand on his chest to indicate 'me'. The staff member said 'Somebody left the door open when they were changing you in the bathroom?' Dominic nodded and looked very upset.

The staff member was able to talk further with Dominic to establish which member of staff had not respected Dominic's privacy. This was then raised directly with the person. All members of staff were reminded that they needed to ensure the same degree of privacy to residents as they would want for themselves. Dominic was satisfied that his complaint had been acted upon.

AAC AND
ACCESS TO
THE WORLD

MULTI-MEDIA AND
ENVIRONMENTAL CONTROL

We might take for granted the ability to 'Google it' and send a quick text message to a loved one. Our phones are multi-media devices allowing us to play music and video and listen to podcasts and audio books.

Computer- and tablet-based AAC solutions have the capacity to incorporate these mainstream apps into the AAC software. From their vocabulary package, AAC users can compose a text message or search instruction, and copy it into an email or search engine.

AAC software developers are finding ways of enabling AAC users to use mainstream software. For example, 'Windows Control' in Jabbla's 'Mind Express' software allows an AAC user to control their computer using their usual access method, be it eye-gaze, switch-scanning or an alternative mouse. They can then access search engines and websites, word-processing and email applications. Accessibility options include magnifying the text or the buttons on the screen, enabling alternative ways of performing mouse functions like a right and left click and drag-and-drop, or of performing touch-screen functions such as a swipe. For AAC users who use switch-scanning, parts of the screen might be highlighted and then selected.

SOCIAL MEDIA

Social media has added a new mode of communication to the world around us. Social media allows us to connect with other people remotely, either with people we know in our everyday lives, or people who we wouldn't otherwise get to interact with. We have the chance to 'find our tribe', connecting with people who share our interests, sense of humour, political views, cultural identifications and so on.

Because social media draws on visual media, it is potentially more accessible to AAC users than a text-only application. However social media platforms develop extremely quickly, and there can be a time-lag between a platform becoming popular, and accessibility options being available on the platform. AAC software developers are often working on a solution, and it may be worth the AAC user making contact with them to discuss their needs.

ENVIRONMENTAL CONTROL

It is possible to allow for a computer or tablet-based AAC device to have integrated environmental controls. This might allow the AAC user to turn lights on or off, open doors, or control their TV, phone or a smart device.

An SLT would not be expected to have a working knowledge of this technology unless they are an AAC specialist working in a regional assessment centre. It is advisable to seek the advice of AAC specialists within your geographical area. Sometimes the Environmental Controls Service is integrated within a regional specialised AAC service, and the AAC user can be assessed holistically for their needs. See Chapter 47 for more information about referring to a specialised AAC assessment centre.

RECOMMENDED RESOURCES

Communication Matters is a UK-based charity for AAC. Every year they host their annual conference which showcases the latest developments in AAC and Assistive Technology (AT). Their website has links for relevant resources, and there is an online discussion group, the AAC Forum, where AAC and AT solutions are often discussed and shared.

AAC COMPETENCIES

Over the last 30 years, AAC expert Janice Light has developed a framework of AAC competencies[1] which are useful when we are setting long-term and short-term goals for an AAC user. These competencies are moving an AAC user towards overall communicative competence.

She sets out four competencies: linguistic, operational, social and strategic.

LINGUISTIC COMPETENCE

This encompasses receptive and expressive language. An AAC user has to understand spoken language, and they have to respond using AAC language.

We are working towards the AAC user understanding and using an expanding vocabulary, made up of core and fringe words. Depending on the AAC user, these words may be represented by symbols or text.

We are working towards them understanding and combining increasing numbers of words to build phrases and sentences. Depending on the AAC user, we may be requiring them to use ready-made phrases, or building a phrase from scratch. We may be working towards them using complex grammar, including negatives, plurals and verb tenses.

Literacy skills feed into linguistic competence, as AAC users develop their use of text-to-speech. They may spell words, use prediction and use pre-made phrases and sentences.

OPERATIONAL COMPETENCE

This takes into account how the AAC user accesses their AAC solution. They may use direct or indirect selection. Direct

DOI: 10.4324/9781003296850-52

selection includes pointing, eye-pointing, using a pointer, using a mouse or a mouse alternative such as a joystick or rollerball, and using eye-gaze technology. Indirect selection includes partner-assisted scanning or switch-scanning.

These access methods each have stages of learning associated with them. It may take time and practice to become proficient. The AAC user will need to learn to scan and select vocabulary, and possibly to find vocabulary across multiple pages. It will take time and practice for them to learn motor patterns that help this process become less effortful and more automatic.

If the AAC user has a computer or tablet-based VOCA, they may need learn how to switch it on and off and adjust settings such as the speech volume. They may need to learn how to use different applications, such as email or text-messaging.

SOCIAL COMPETENCE

This begins with developing communicative intent, joint attention and using non-verbal communication to add to a given message. It involves being able to give a consistent 'yes' or 'no' response. It also includes the skill of taking turns in a conversation, and how to initiate or end or maintain conversation.

We are working towards an AAC user being able to express a range of communication functions, including requesting, commenting, describing, asking and answering questions. Ultimately we may be aiming for an AAC user to be able to convey their thoughts and feelings and move beyond the 'here-and-now' to tell real and imagined stories, talk about past events and project into the future.

STRATEGIC COMPETENCE

AAC communication has many challenges, and the AAC user must learn how to communicate in a speaking world. This may include a way of communicating that they use AAC. They may need to use a communication passport to explain their needs. They may have a wrist band that they hold up to request their AAC system. They may learn to use quick phrases to explain their needs, for example, 'please wait whilst I type a message'. They may have access to 'floor-holding' phrases like 'uh-huh'.

The AAC user will sometimes need to use quick telegraphic messages as opposed to complete sentences. For example, 'Stop! Not that!' They may need to use repair strategies, for example when they can't find the right word on their AAC system, they might say 'it's similar to' or 'I will try to spell it'.

The AAC user will need to judge which mode of communication is best suited to a given situation. Sometimes they may choose to use their communication book, whilst at other times they may choose their VOCA.

PSYCHOSOCIAL FACTORS

In addition to these four competencies, Light describes psychosocial factors which support successful use of AAC.

The AAC user needs *motivation* in order to persist in learning these diverse skills for AAC communication.

They will have to draw on a positive and persevering *attitude*, because there will be barriers to their successful communication.

They will need to build *confidence* in communicating first with supportive communication partners and then unfamiliar communication partners.

A certain amount of *resilience* is also necessary, for example if the AAC system fails, or if communication partners are not supportive.

ENVIRONMENTAL SUPPORTS AND BARRIERS

It is an incomplete picture to only focus upon the AAC user. Conversations are co-created between the AAC user and their communication partners. The conversation partner may be more or less attuned to the AAC user, creating either opportunities for richer shared meaning, or restricting the AAC user's potential. As SLTs, we need to work with communication partners just as much as the AAC user (see Chapters 11 and 12).

The AAC user operates within a society that frequently misunderstands and underestimates their abilities. The SLT, the AAC user or the AAC user's advocate may need to undertake some wider awareness work to inform schools, workplaces and the community about AAC and AAC users.

A recent development in the UK is the launch of a blue 'Communication Access Symbol' to build awareness of the needs of people with communication difficulties. It is the equivalent of the familiar blue signs for supporting people with visual impairment or hearing impairment that we see in public places and organisations. Organisations can sign up to a brief training session, which covers strategies like giving a person time to communicate, listening carefully and observing their multi-modal communication. The organisation is then registered as communication friendly and can display the Communication Access Symbol.

Under the Equality Act 2010, education settings and workplaces have to allow reasonable adjustments for those with disabilities. Funding is available for individuals and organisations to purchase necessary equipment to allow a person to access education or do their job.

A recent development is 'job-crafting',[2] where a job can be matched to the needs of the individual. An agency might assist this process. This gets away from the idea that the individual must be perfect before applying for a job. Instead it utilises a concept of 'sheltered employment' whereby the employer and colleagues can nurture the individual, so that they acquire a social identity and gain professional competencies in the role.

An SLT needs to be aware of these initiatives so that they can signpost an individual to the support they need.

RECOMMENDED RESOURCES

The Augmentative and Alternative Communication Profile by Tracy Kovach is an assessment tool which can be used to profile an AAC user's current competencies. This can then inform areas to be targeted in interventions.

Informal conversations around the competencies outlined above may be enough to inform objectives. It is likely that the

AAC user and their communication partner will have a good idea of where communication is falling down.

The next chapter will consider objective setting.

NOTES

1 Light, J. and McNaughton, D. 'Communicative competence for individuals who require augmentative and alternative communication: a new definition for a new era of communication?' *Augmentative and Alternative Communication*, 2014, 30(1).

2 Scopetta, A., Daverne, E and Geyer, L. 'Job carving and job crafting: a review of practices', European Commission, 2019.

SETTING OBJECTIVES

The AAC competencies outlined in the previous chapter may be used to shape objectives for a specific AAC user and their communication partners. The table below gives examples of possible objectives within each area of competence. This list is by no means exhaustive: it gives a flavour of possible objectives. The SLT can adapt these to meet the needs of an individual AAC user.

Objectives should be set collaboratively with the AAC user and their communication partners. This way, they will be signed up to the work ahead.

I haven't included the psychosocial factors in these suggestions for objectives. This is because shifts in an AAC user's motivation, attitudes, confidence and resilience are hard to prescribe. If the SLT feels that these are issues for the AAC user, then a conversation may be needed to start to probe their significance. A Talking Mat may be useful here (see Chapter 41). This will help guide any actions. An SLT may need to signpost an AAC user to counselling or other forms of psychosocial support around their situation.

If there is insufficient support for an AAC user, then the SLT may provide information or training for a particular setting. The SLT may choose to set an objective around environmental supports and barriers, and I have included suggestions below.

LINGUISTIC COMPETENCE

- The AAC user will explore the vocabulary contained within specific pages of their communication book.

 DOI: 10.4324/9781003296850-53

- The AAC user will combine core and fringe words to create multi-word utterances.
- The AAC user will begin to use grammatical morphemes, including plural –s.
- The AAC user will begin to select the correct verb tense when they are using their vocabulary package on their VOCA.
- The AAC user will use their alphabet chart to start to spell words.

OPERATIONAL COMPETENCE

- The AAC user will visually scan all of the symbols on a page before making their selection.
- The AAC user will indicate 'yes' by nodding when the communication partner reads out the options in their partner-assisted auditory scanning book.
- The AAC user will turn to the relevant page of their communication book independently.
- The AAC user will turn the VOCA on or off as needed.

SOCIAL COMPETENCE

- The AAC user will greet their friends when they arrive for the conversation group.
- The AAC user will maintain the topic of conversation for two to three turns.
- The AAC user will begin to answer questions in group time.
- The AAC user will give their opinion about the SLT session using their AAC system.

STRATEGIC COMPETENCE

- The AAC user will initiate communication by holding up their wristband which says 'I have something to say'.
- The AAC user will use their communication board to communicate when their VOCA is on charge.

- The AAC user will use telegraphic messages using core words for urgent care needs, e.g. 'no more' or 'it here'.
- The AAC user will indicate when the communication partner has misunderstood their message.

ENVIRONMENTAL SUPPORTS AND BARRIERS

- The teaching team will consistently get out the communication board at the start of the school day.
- The conversation partner will model two-word phrases using core words.
- The care staff will use the visual support for communication menu options each day.
- The conversation partner will read through the options on the partner-assisted auditory scanning communication book, waiting for the AAC user to indicate 'yes'.
- The AAC user's partner will position the eye-gaze device as shown in their communication passport.

THERAPY OUTCOME MEASURES FOR AAC

Therapy Outcome Measures (TOMS), developed by Professor Pam Enderby, can be used to measure the effectiveness of a team's therapy interventions. In the AAC scale, SLTs can match an individual to a detailed description of their impairment (be it physical, sensory, cognitive or speech and language), the communication support for that person, the communication activities they are able to undertake, their participation in different social roles and their overall wellbeing. These domains are assessed again after the intervention period.

It is recommended that the whole team undertake training on TOMS in order to effectively implement TOMS as an outcome measure. There are many other scales in addition to AAC, including for Developmental Language Disorder, Dysarthria and Aphasia.

FUNDING FOR AAC

SPECIALIST AAC ASSESSMENT

LOCAL SLT SERVICES

The majority of people who require AAC in the UK will have their needs met by their local SLT services.

SLTs who work in local services will provide advice about paper-based AAC solutions, single- or multiple-message VOCAs, basic AAC apps and directly accessed text-to-speech AAC solutions. They may support the process of message-banking or voice-banking for those with rapidly degenerating conditions. Local commissioning arrangements will be in place to provide equipment to support this work.

Within local services, the local SLT may seek support from a more experienced colleague, or a colleague who has a special interest in AAC.

If an individual has complex access needs and paper-based AAC is not meeting their needs, then the local SLT may consider referring to a specialised AAC service.

SPECIALISED AAC SERVICES

The UK has commissioning arrangements in place to provide access to specialist AAC assessment for those who need it. There is broad consistency between England, Scotland, Wales and Northern Ireland in terms of eligibility criteria.

The eligibility criteria for NHSE, updated in 2021, is that an individual must:

- have a severe or complex communication difficulty associated with a range of physical or cognitive impairments.

If sensory deficits exist, these are not the primary cause for the communication need.

- are able to understand the purpose of a communication aid.
- have developed beyond basic cause-and-effect understanding.
- are able to understand the purpose of a communication aid.
- have a clear discrepancy between their understanding of language and their ability to use natural speech.
- have experience of using paper-based AAC which is insufficient to enable them to meet their communication potential.
- have demonstrated that they can learn how to use paper-based AAC, with examples given of how this has enabled them to convey a range of communication functions.
- If the person is using the alphabet to compose AAC messages, their physical needs mean that they require an alternative access method.

If the answer to any of these questions is 'no', then the person's AAC needs will be met by local services. Other support and funding streams for equipment may also be considered (see the following chapter).

People with rapidly degenerating conditions, such as Motor Neurone Disease, can be referred before they meet all of the above criteria. They do not need to wait until their speech or hand function has deteriorated.

PRE-REFERRAL WORK

The local SLT will have worked with the individual to assess their language and AAC needs (see Chapter 5). They may have explored paper-based AAC, and possibly single- or multiple-message VOCAs or apps on a mainstream tablet.

The AAC solutions tried so far are inadequate to meet the individual's ongoing communication needs. This may be because they cannot access the solution using conventional direct selection, like pointing or pressing a button with their finger. It may be because the AAC solution does not give them access to enough vocabulary or allow them to combine words or symbols into complex messages conveying a range of communication functions.

The local SLT will need to help gather information about how the individual is using their current AAC solution, and what has been tried. This may take the form of video evidence, or transcriptions of their communication messages.

Ideally, the SLT will make a referral to specialised AAC services collaboratively with the AAC user, their family, and other professionals who are involved with the AAC user. It is very helpful for an OT or physiotherapist to add information about the individual's fine or gross motor skills and any equipment they use, including wheelchairs or seating systems. If the referral is for a child or young person, then their teacher will need to be involved. It is helpful for the specialist AAC assessment service to know the child's literacy levels, so that they can consider how to support the child with the alphabet or text-to-speech.

THE ASSESSMENT

Once an individual is accepted for assessment, further information about their needs may be gathered. There may be an assessment planning meeting with the person and the team around them. A specialist assessment will usually be carried out by a specialist SLT, and is likely to also include an OT, healthcare scientist or clinical technologist. Some AAC assessment centres also have specialist teachers.

An assessment will usually be face-to-face, involving the person trying out computer- or tablet-based VOCAs and possibly different access methods.

If a person's access needs are very complex, there may be a short trial period of an AAC solution, to try to get the 'best fit' solution. There will inevitably be some compromises as the team balances out the person's visual, physical and communication needs. There are frequently factors around positioning and fatigue, the communication environment, and the current capability of technology solutions.

Once the 'best fit' solution has been determined, the individual will receive a long-term loan of the device. The assessment centre will advise on who to contact for maintenance or breakage issues. Most assessment centres will offer training or support for the initial implementation of the AAC solution.

The individual will then be passed back to local services for ongoing support. This may take the form of setting communication objectives for the individual and their communication partners. There will be local commissioning arrangements for how this support is to be provided.

MENTORING OR TRAINING

Some specialised AAC assessment centres may be able to offer training for local SLTs so that they can develop their expertise in this area.

If a person is accepted for assessment, then the local SLT will be involved in this process. They have important knowledge about the individual, and will be key in supporting with the implementation of an AAC solution.

The SLT, AAC user and their family will be learning together. A key skill in AAC implementation is the willingness to make mistakes. The SLT can model this for the AAC user. AAC is generally 'trial-and-error': we only get to the 'best fit' solution by having a go.

If you are an SLT with an interest in this field, then ask about mentoring or shadowing opportunities at your nearest AAC assessment centre. See also Chapter 50 for more information on CPD.

REASSESSMENT

AAC devices do not last forever, and it is likely that a computer- or tablet-based VOCA will begin to fail after several years of use. The local SLT may need to re-refer to a specialised AAC centre for reassessment.

If the AAC user's needs have not changed, then the SLT may request a 'like-for-like' replacement, as an equipment-only request. However, if the AAC user's needs have changed, in terms of their physical, sensory, cognitive or communication needs, then they may have a full assessment for a new device.

RECOMMENDED RESOURCES

See the 'Communication Matters' website for up-to-date information about specialised AAC assessment in the UK. The website lists all of the specialised services, with links to referral information.

OTHER FUNDING STREAMS

There will be times when an individual does not meet the criteria for funding for an AAC device from statutory services. In this case, they may choose to pursue alternative sources of funding.

CHARITABLE FUNDING

The Sequal Trust has a long history of funding communication devices for those people who do not meet NHS criteria. They can provide different types of VOCA, from multiple message VOCAs to tablet- and computer-based solutions.

Find a Voice is a national charity which can loan out communication devices for a period of time. This might inform a funding application to purchase a device.

Charities which support a particular condition may offer a loan bank of equipment or funding for equipment. The MND Association and Muscular Dystrophy UK both have schemes. The Children's Trust supports children with brain injury. Just4Children, Lifeline4Kids and the Aidis Trust support children with disabilities.

The Family Fund and Family Welfare Association can support with funding for families on a low income.

PRIVATE FUNDING

The ACE Centre can provide independent AAC assessments for those people who do not meet NHS criteria.

ASLTIP (Association of Speech and Language Therapists in Independent Practice) have some SLTs who are able to assess for AAC solutions. It is recommended that they work in partnership with an OT where AAC users have complex access needs.

DOI: 10.4324/9781003296850-56

A BUSINESS CASE FOR AAC RESOURCES

A business case is a formal written document submitted to those who approve funding for a service initiative, including equipment and resources. A good business case will be concise, specific and factual. It will use reliable sources of data, including clinical populations and costs.

The business case will state the benefit to the clinical population served. It may demonstrate the cost effectiveness or time effectiveness of this initiative, in contrast with current arrangements. This may include the sustainability over time. It may reference clinical guidelines or research evidence in support of the proposal. It may include any data collected to support the clinical effectiveness of the initiative.

The business case will also state what is required from all stakeholders, in terms of finances and time. It will factor in any staff time and training and support from other departments such as admin and IT. It may include how this initiative promotes joined-up care between health, education and social care, or how it promotes the current service improvement plan.

SBAR

A tool used in the NHS for allowing prompt and appropriate communication is an SBAR. SBAR stands for Situation, Background, Assessment and Recommendation.

This may prove a useful tool to building a business case for AAC resources. Below is a suggested outline which may be adapted for your particular needs.

DOI: 10.4324/9781003296850-57

SITUATION

The SLT service currently holds ageing stock of AAC resources and software, which is inadequate for the clinical population.

The service currently has a caseload of [number of people]. It is estimated that [number] would benefit from some form of AAC, including visual supports, communication boards and books.

Research into clinical populations across the UK[1] and NHSE guidance for commissioning AAC services[2] and equipment estimates that 0.05% of the population require AAC. Local SLT services should meet the needs of 90% of these people, with the remaining 10% requiring referral to specialised AAC assessment services. This proposal supports the adequate resourcing of local services in order to fulfil local commissioning arrangements and allow for appropriate referral to regional specialised services.

The provision of appropriate AAC has an impact upon an individual's health and wellbeing and their access to work and education. AAC allows users to be effectively consulted about their needs and choices with regards to health, education and social care provision.

BACKGROUND

The SLT service has minimally invested in AAC resources in recent years.

The software used to create paper-based symbolised supports, including communication boards and books, is now over five years old. It is extremely glitchy, and frequently freezes, meaning that work is lost. This means that making resources takes at least twice as long as it needs to.

The team has accessed a free trial of Widgit Online software for 1 month during November. This allowed us to make AAC resources to meet the needs of 23 people in this time period.

Widgit Online allows sharing of resources to minimise reduplication of effort within the service. There is a significant time saving when staff can access premade templates of communication books and boards and overlays for multiple message devices such as the SuperTalker and GoTalk. Thus, a resource which currently takes an hour to produce on our outdated software takes less than ten minutes to produce using current software. There is an impact upon staff motivation and satisfaction, as evidenced in the recent NHS staff survey.

We have collected feedback from service users and 94% of responses rated the AAC resources provided as 'extremely useful' or 'very useful' (with other options being 'somewhat useful' and 'not useful'. 92% of service users said that they either used these AAC resources 'every day' or 'several times a week' (with other options being 'once per week' or 'less than once per week'.

In terms of hardware, the SLT service has very few AAC devices which are functioning properly. Our current stock consists of two Big Macks, a SuperTalker and a GoTalk 20+ and a GoTalk 32+. This is not adequate for the caseload. There are not enough devices to be trialled with the people who need them.

AAC technology has moved on rapidly in recent years, with AAC apps now being available on iPads. This is an extremely effective way to trial an AAC solution in preparation for referring service-users to the specialised AAC assessment service.

ASSESSMENT

Based on current caseload figures and the number of SLTs in our service, we estimate that we require the following resources.

Item	Cost per item
Widgit Online Group Account	
2 Big Macks	
1 iTalk 2 with levels	
SuperTalker FT	
GoTalk 20+	
Go Talk 32+	
5 iPads	
5 Grid for iPad apps	
5 rugged cases for iPads	

RECOMMENDATION

It is recommended that these items are purchased in this year's budget. The Widgit Online group account will need to be factored in each year's budget planning. It is estimated that the BigMacks, iTalk 2, SuperTalker and Go Talks will have a life of more than ten years, based on previous purchases. The iPads are likely to need replacing in five to seven years.

We will continue to use a colour printer with replaceable ink cartridges, and a laminator. These ongoing costs are already factored into the budget.

The SLT service will require support from IT to set up the iPads with the required apps. The iPads will need to be managed to be compliant with current GDPR regulations. Admin will need to support a booking process to ensure that iPads are effectively shared throughout the team.

It is suggested that all SLT staff attend free eLearning training provided from our specialised AAC assessment service. Training is available both for using the Widgit Online software and trialling and apps on iPads. Each of these eLearning modules takes 30 minutes to complete. It will be a requirement for SLTs to have attended this before they can book out equipment.

The service will continue to closely monitor service user feedback about the quality and effectiveness of AAC resources supplied. The service will also seek feedback from the specialised AAC assessment service and Social Care Services about the resources being supplied.

NOTES

1 Communication Matters, 'Shining a Light on Augmentative and Alternative Communication' final report, 2013.
2 NHSE, 'Guidance for Commissioning AAC Services and Equipment', 2016.

CONTINUING PROFESSIONAL DEVELOPMENT

SLTs have a responsibility to keep up to date with evidence-based practice. Below are suggestions for sources of information and inspiration in AAC practice.

COURSES

Regional specialised AAC assessment services are commissioned to provide training and support for local services. This may take the form of face-to-face or remote training, or eLearning modules. These may be free or chargeable.

ELEARNING

Kent and Medway Communication and Assistive Technology (KM CAT) offer a suite of eLearning training modules, which are free to anyone. Modules include moving a child beyond requesting, the skills needed for eye-gaze, and teaching literacy to non-verbal children.

There are two excellent sites which have extensive eLearning modules focused towards the North American context, but applicable to other countries. 'Project Core' is all about implementation of AAC, focusing on a 'Universal Core' of 38 core words which can be used in any situation. The eLearning modules are accompanied by free downloadable AAC resources featuring the universal core words. 'Dynamic Learning Maps' is linked with Karen Erickson's work, and has a suite of eLearning modules to support teaching literacy to children with complex needs. These two sites may be overwhelming if you are new to AAC, but are excellent for a developing specialist.

DOI: 10.4324/9781003296850-58

WEBSITES

Communication Matters is the UK chapter of ISAAC, The International Society for Augmentative and Alternative Communication. Both have websites which have information about all things AAC. Both organisations offer annual conferences where AAC users and experts from around the world give presentations around current research and best clinical practice.

Communication Matters has an AAC Forum for AAC users, families and professionals, where people post queries about AAC solutions and interventions. This is a great way to ask clinical questions and share ideas.

The ACE Centre and CALL Scotland have excellent websites full of information and free downloadable resources.

JOURNALS

Augmentative and Alternative Communication is the official journal of ISAAC and publishes quarterly. Occasional papers on AAC also appear in the *International Journal of Language Communication Disorders*, the *Journal of Speech, Hearing and Language Research*, the *International Journal of Speech-Language Pathology*, the *Journal of Developmental and Physical Disabilities* and *Seminars in Speech and Language*.

BOOKS

The classic AAC text book is Beukelman and Light's *Augmentative and Alternative Communication: Supporting Children and Adults with Complex Communication Needs*. It covers assessment and intervention, including a range of AAC solutions and access methods. It also covers AAC competencies, as set out by Janice Light.

Highly recommended is Erna Alant's *Augmentative and Alternative Communication: Engagement and Participation*. This is not so much a guide to AAC options, as a philosophical and practical treatise on promoting shared creation of meaning for genuine connection and rich relationships.

A UK-specific book is the author's *Who's Afraid of AAC?: The UK Guide to Augmentative and Alternative Communication*. This is an in-depth practical guide for assessment and implementation across the lifespan, intended for parents and carers as well as health, education and social care professionals. All pages, including activities and ideas, are photocopiable.

BLOGS AND SOCIAL MEDIA

These are dynamic, fast-paced sources of personal stories, inspiration and opinions. They are often from the AAC user or a family member's perspective, so give an insight into real-life challenges and triumphs. #seemeseemyaac has been a successful campaign across social media platforms where videos and photos have been posted to show everyday use of AAC.

There are also some sites specifically aimed at professionals. PrAACtical AAC is an excellent site which showcases the best in AAC implementation.

EMAIL LISTS

Communication Matters releases a weekly news bulletin each Friday. This lists any training or events offered by specialised AAC assessment services or AAC suppliers, as well as the CM annual conference and any smaller events they may be organising. There are also opportunities to contribute to research projects in the field of AAC.

Other AAC organisations, including Makaton, Widgit and the main AAC suppliers, offer the option to sign up to their email lists. They send regular updates about resources, products, training or media campaigns.

BIBLIOGRAPHY

BOOKS

The classic AAC text book is Beukelman and Light's *Augmentative and Alternative Communication: Supporting Children and Adults with Complex Communication Needs*. It covers assessment and intervention, including a range of AAC solutions and access methods. It also covers AAC competencies, as set out by Janice Light.

Highly recommended is Erna Alant's *Augmentative and Alternative Communication: Engagement and Participation*. This is not so much a guide to AAC options, as a philosophical and practical treatise on promoting shared creation of meaning for genuine connection and rich relationships.

A UK-specific book is the author's *Who's Afraid of AAC?: The UK Guide to Augmentative and Alternative Communication*. This is an in-depth practical guide for assessment and implementation across the lifespan, intended for parents and carers as well as health, education and social care professionals. All pages, including activities and ideas, are photocopiable.

INDEX

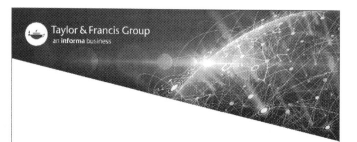

Printed in the United States
by Baker & Taylor Publisher Services